# Toward a Science of Psychiatry

## Impact of the Research Development Program of the National Institute of Mental Health

# Toward a Science of Psychiatry

## Impact of the Research Development Program of the National Institute of Mental Health

Bert E. Boothe
Anne H. Rosenfeld
Edward L. Walker

Brooks/Cole Publishing Company
Monterey, California

A Division of Wadsworth Publishing Company, Inc.

ISBN: 0-8185-0107-3
L.C. Catalog Card No.: 73-87501
Printed in the United States of America
1 2 3 4 5 6 7 8 9 10—78 77 76 75 74

Production Editor: Mara Niels
Interior & Cover Design: Linda Marcetti
Typesetting: The Heffernan Press, Inc., Worcester, Massachusetts
Printing & Binding: The Colonial Press, Inc., Clinton, Massachusetts

# Foreword

## John Romano

For some time before his death, Bert E. Boothe had planned to write a report describing the design and progress of the Research Development Program of the National Institute of Mental Health. Edward L. Walker and Anne H. Rosenfeld have completed his project, *Toward a Science of Psychiatry* describes the success of the Research Development Program in effecting a significant change in the number and quality of psychiatrists and others interested and engaged in sustained investigative work in psychiatry. Certain chapters of this book have special historical value—such as Chapter 4 on psychoanalysis, which, although born in Europe, flourished as a particularly American experience. Other chapters give a clear account of the development of ideas and hypotheses from the several belief systems that contribute today to the understanding of the mentally sick person, his family, and his community. The final chapter and the appendices will be useful to present and future historians in recording the growth and development of psychiatric research in the past 25 years.

During the mid-1940s, those of us associated with the Research Study Section of NIMH soon became aware of the scarcity of young men and women engaged significantly in psychiatric research. It became clear that the field needed a new type of psychiatrist—namely, the research scientist, as contrasted with the teacher-clinician, the practicing psychiatrist, the psychotherapist, or the administrative officer. Unlike our colleagues in medicine and physiology, we in psychiatry did not have a Rockefeller Institute to help prepare young men and women for pro-

John Romano, M. D., is Distinguished University Professor of Psychiatry at the University of Rochester School of Medicine and Dentistry, Rochester, New York.

fessorial posts and research careers. Before 1946, when few persons were engaged in investigative work, appropriate models for the young to emulate were rarely found. Earlier in the century, whatever research had been conducted was done under private auspices or in a few large state mental hospitals. Support subsequently came from state funds through the development of the Psychopathic Hospital movement in Ann Arbor, Iowa City, Denver, and Boston. Contributions were made by the Rockefeller Foundation, the Scottish Rite, and the Commonwealth Fund.

Given this background, one can understand the excitement and promise of the Congressional action that established the National Mental Health Law in 1946. By the late 1940s, we were fortunate that two recently created programs for supporting research scientists—The Markle Scholarship in Medicine, founded in 1948, and the American Heart Association's Lifetime Career Award—met needs similar to ours. We used these two as models to guide us in drafting proposals for the Career Investigator Grant Awards in psychiatry.

For about 10 years before he came to NIMH in 1957, Bert and I had corresponded, principally exchanging information about candidates for the Menninger School of Psychiatry; a number of these candidates had been my students at Harvard, Cincinnati, and Rochester. Bert and I subsequently had an opportunity to work together when he succeeded Philip Sapir as the Executive Secretary of the Mental Health Career Investigator Selection Committee at NIMH. In his devotion and commitment to this position, he was extraordinarily useful in helping the Committee make important judgments about the selection of promising young scientists in our field. He joined us at Arden House at the first meeting of the young investigators and was the principal planner and engineer of subsequent annual meetings. (Incidentally, we are again indebted to the Markle Scholarship Plan for the idea of convening our investigators. The Markle group had done this successfully for a number of years before our first meeting.)

Over the years, Bert became a truly charismatic figure to those young men and women who had been recipients of Career Investigator and Research Career Development awards. They found him to be an able, intelligent, thoughtful, and always helpful person. They recognized that his interest in them was genuine and sustained, and he was both fatherly and motherly in doing much to help them in their later careers. He was modest, even shy at times, gentle, and most generous of himself and in his work with others.

I am sure that the success of this report stems from the thoughtful candor of the many respondents quoted throughout it. The quality and extent of this response is a function of the awardees' respect, admiration, and affection for Bert Boothe.

# Foreword

## Philip Sapir

Luckily, there are men and women of dedication and imagination whose presence and actions make a difference in whether programs succeed or fail, are carried out with strength and grace or bumble along in traditional bureaucratic fashion.

Bert E. Boothe was such a dedicated man—one who believed that the betterment of man can result only from understanding his strengths and weaknesses and their sources; that such understanding lies within the domain of psychiatry and the behavioral sciences generally; and that to further such understanding and its application it is necessary to seek out and encourage able, sensitive, and creative investigators.

In his work as program director of the Research Development Program of NIMH, Bert had a deep, abiding concern for the well-being and advancement of those who sought and received the program's support and those who graduated from the program to positions of responsibility and honor. Although he was interested in the nature, quality, and progress of their research undertakings, he was concerned more broadly with their development as individuals and scholars who, by deepening their sensitivities to human needs and problems, would not only become better people themselves but also ultimately contribute more to the field. Bert's interest in the welfare of these individual scientists became a lifetime concern. That concern was reciprocated by the deep respect and fondness that the awardees had for him. They turned to him often for advice and support during difficult times and at decision points in their careers. Beyond the personal significance to grantees of Bert's dedication,

Philip Sapir is the Director of The Grant Foundation, Inc.

his presence, sensibility, and fortitude contributed significantly to the impact this program has had.

The program has established the reality and practicality of pursuing a lifetime career in psychiatric and behavioral research in this country; however, this accomplishment may be evanescent. The current ominous trends in the cutback of federal support of science and of institutions of higher education bode ill for programs such as these. An unfortunate concomitant of earlier federal largesse in the support of science has been the development of an attitude in universities and colleges that support of science is the proper concern primarily of government and not these institutions themselves, which now see their role as transmitting existing knowledge, not advancing it. With clinical practice, psychotherapy, community mental health practice, and administration offering the lures of greater financial rewards, security, and prestige, it is possible that this recently established discipline of research psychiatry will become once again the province of only a few dedicated individuals and institutions. Add to this the current legitimate concern for the expanded and improved delivery of health services and the belief that research is not the concern of state and local government, and it is not difficult to see why some of us fear for the future.

It is not enough to reiterate that the ultimate cure of disease lies in the development of new knowledge. Our field has a twofold responsibility: we must develop new knowledge in the hope of ultimately curing disease; at the same time, we must also apply existing knowledge to improving health care for all. We must re-evaluate how the academic venture—including its education, training, research, and service aspects—can be encouraged and related productively to other societal ventures in government, business, community agencies and services, and private philanthropy. Meager as the practical results of psychiatric and behavioral research to date may be, we must hope for recognition of the need to develop, sustain, and support a continuing flow of fresh talent to tackle the most challenging problem of this and all times—the proper growth, development, and nurturance of the human mind and spirit.

# Acknowledgments

Many people have helped in creating this book—far too many to list—but the following individuals and organizations have made indispensable contributions: Philip Sapir of The Grant Foundation; O. Meredith Wilson and Preston Cutler of the Center for Advanced Studies in the Behavioral Sciences; Research Development Program Committee members David A. Hamburg, Daniel X. Freedman, Ernest A. Haggard, Albert J. Silverman, Samuel Eiduson, Akira Horita, Joseph C. Speisman, Albert J. Stunkard, Alberta E. Siegel, Lucy Rau Ferguson, Herbert Weiner; Research Development Program awardees past and present; Mary R. Haworth, Betty H. Pickett, Louis A. Wienckowski, David Shakow, John E. Eberhardt, and Halvor Rosvold, of the National Institute of Mental Health; and other NIMH staff who provided information, checked for scientific and historical accuracy, and aided in producing the final manuscript; chairmen of departments of psychiatry throughout the country, including Frederick C. Redlich; staff members of the Center for Advanced Studies in the Behavioral Sciences, including Carol Treanor, Jane Kielsmeier, Nancy B. Helmy, and Susan Custer; typists Elizabeth Armour and Val Faulkenburg; and Mara Niels, Charles T. Hendrix, and other staff members of Brooks/Cole Publishing Company who have made this book possible.

Our special thanks go to Helvi Boothe, who helped translate Bert's intentions into a published volume.

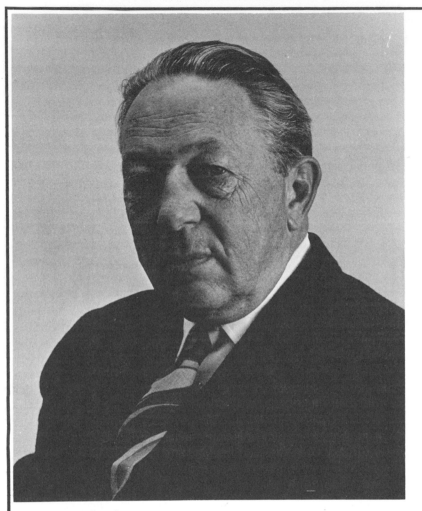

*Bert Edwin Boothe*

# Dedicated to
# Bert Edwin Boothe
# 1906-1972

Bert E. Boothe was born in Sumner, Michigan, on July 1, 1906. After receiving a Bachelor's degree from Central State Teacher's College at Mt. Pleasant, Michigan, in 1925, he became an English teacher at Grand Marais High School in Grand Marais, Michigan. He attended the summer session at Columbia University in 1926 and within a year became Principal of the high school in Sparta, Michigan. In 1929 he returned to graduate study in Renaissance literature and taught English at the University of Michigan. He took the Master's degree in 1930 and the Ph.D. in 1936. During a brief career in the academic world, he was Assistant Professor of English at Iowa State Teacher's College at Cedar Falls, Iowa, for two years and served as head of the department for an additional two years. He then became Professor of English at Chicago Teacher's College and Assistant Editor of *College English*.

Boothe's academic career was jolted onto an entirely new course by his military service. Entering the Army in 1943, he was assigned to the Information and Education Office in San Juan, Puerto Rico. When his military service ended, he was invited by Dr. Karl Menninger to the Menninger Foundation in Topeka, Kansas, where he served for a year as Assistant Director of the Department of Education. When the Menninger School of Psychiatry was formed in 1946, he became Director of Professional Education in the Veterans Administration Hospital in Topeka, Kansas, which was affiliated with that school. There he was responsible for developing an extensive psychiatric residency program that he integrated with training programs in clinical psychology, psychiatric social work, and psychiatric nursing. In this position, he earned the Outstanding Performance Award from the Veterans Administration in 1956 and in 1957.

Boothe moved to Washington in 1957 to become Administrator of the Fellowship and Career Investigator Grant Programs of the National Institute of Mental Health (NIMH). Four years later, in 1961, he became Chief of the Research Fellowships Section of the Research Grants Branch. (In 1964, the Research Fellowships Section was shifted to the Training and Manpower Resources Branch.) In 1968, he became Chief of the Behavioral Sciences Training Branch.

Boothe became a Fellow of the Center for Advanced Study in the Behavioral Sciences in 1971 and was in residence at the Center at the time of his death on June 5, 1972.

# Contents

# Introduction

Psychiatry, long an art, is becoming a science as well. Significant in this transformation has been the Research Development Program[1] of the National Institute of Mental Health, which for 20 years has supported talented psychiatrists and biobehavioral scientists as they train for and engage in careers in psychiatric research. *Toward a Science of Psychiatry* examines—largely from the perspective of the scientist-grantees, administrators, and advisors who have had contact with the Research Development Program—the progress of psychiatric research during the past two decades and the program's role in bringing this progress about.

Bert E. Boothe conceived the purpose of this book as follows:

> I begin with some assumptions: that the past 20 years have produced most of the research development that has occurred in psychiatry; that the work of people who have had some support from the NIMH Career Investigator Grant program (and the later Research Career Award and Research Scientist Development programs) has been significant and representative in psychiatric research; and that, therefore, by explaining accomplishments associated with these, one can say something useful about psychiatric research.

Psychiatry has not gained its emergent status as a science easily. Its lack of a research tradition has reflected a set of attitudes in the pro-

---

[1] Because the program has undergone a number of name changes over the years, the term "Research Development Program" will be used to encompass the entire program from 1954 to the present; the term "Research Scientist Development Program" refers specifically to the most recent form of the program, from 1967 to the present.

fession that have often valued authority over investigation and clinical intuition over experimental proof. Before the 1950s, other fields of medicine were already encouraging and rewarding the research scientist, while psychiatry, for the most part, was not (although of course there have always been some researchers of singular talent attracted to the study of mental illness, its causes, prevention, and treatment).

Since its inception in 1954, the Research Development Program has been notably successful in attracting scientists to psychiatric research despite a tradition in the profession that has stressed and preferentially rewarded clinical skills and orientation. The program's success reflects the sensitivity of its initiators and administrators in choosing appropriate candidates and sponsoring institutions and in designing a program that compensates for many of the hardships of pioneering through adequate incentives—an opportunity for individualized research training, relatively long periods of support (5 to 15 or more years), an adequate salary for full-time research (with no necessity for extra administrative, teaching, or clinical responsibilities), and a degree of honor and status conferred by virtue of the program's exacting, personalized screening process. *Toward a Science of Psychiatry* examines in detail the impact of these provisions on the grantees, their institutions, and the field of psychiatry. This book also discusses some of the chronic problems that have haunted program administrators and grantees: these problems include the difficulty of assuring long-term, continuous support to individuals by a federal agency that inevitably must respond to changes in administrations and national priorities; the hard task of creating a positive climate for research and researchers while coping with the often-strained marriage of convenience between the federal government and the universities; and the challenge of trying to accelerate needed social change without imposing undue hardship on the vanguard—in this case, the program's grantees.

This volume appropriately raises many more questions than it answers. It describes some of the recent past of psychiatric research and sets the stage for an examination of the consequences of this past for the present and future. The experiences of the program and its grantees, deriving from a unique and exciting period for the growth of research, should suggest principles for stimulating further creative research wherever and whenever new knowledge is actively sought.

Despite the progress of the past few decades, psychiatric research is still in its infancy; it is only beginning to develop the theoretical and factual base needed for an effective and humanely scientific branch of medicine. The task before psychiatry remains awesome. Defined narrowly, it is to understand all illnesses of mind and make men well. Defined broadly, it is to discover and enhance the conditions—biological, social, and psychological—that encourage man's fullest development. Taking even the narrow definition, the task looks overwhelming. There have been theories and discoveries and "eras of enlightenment," but we still must search for cures for many of the major forms of mental illness. We are likely to have none in the foreseeable future. Each new flare of discovery has further illuminated the territory of the brain and behavior, but our growing sophistication reveals our ignorance as well; the more we understand, the more there is to understand. The arduous search continues nonetheless, and, in the process, a cadre of talented individuals has brought a new spirit of inquiry into the field, sharpening and seeking answers to many important questions that until recently were not even asked. In Chapter 2, next, the striking range and substance of these questions will be examined.

# The Substance
# of Research

What is psychiatric research? In an effort to answer this question, Chapter 2 will present an overview of the character, flavor, and range of psychiatric research projects conducted by 169 participants in the Research Development Program who have been working in psychiatric settings. To the degree that the interests of these outstanding men and women are representative of all psychiatric researchers, this summary gives a picture not only of their work but of the major directions of psychiatric research over the past two decades.

In keeping with the comprehensive approach of its sponsoring agency, the National Institute of Mental Health, the Research Development Program has taken a broad view of psychiatric research. It has supported scientists pursuing a striking array of mental-health-related problems with varied techniques and orientations. Grantees' research interests include normal and abnormal behavioral and biological functioning studied both in laboratory and clinical settings. Their disciplines run the gamut from biochemistry and psychopharmacology through neurophysiology and psychology to sociology and anthropology. By encouraging this diversity, the ultimate goal of the Research Development Program has become more tangible: to provide a scientific base for psychiatry by understanding the biological, social, and environmental factors that underlie and affect man's mental life and to discover the most effective methods to encourage healthy mental development throughout the life cycle.

Given the wide scope of psychiatric research, no brief treatment such as this can do justice to its range, and few authors' scholarship is sufficiently broad to describe such heterogeneity adequately. So, this book will describe only major trends of the research; it will present quotations from program participants (who answered a questionnaire sent by Dr. Boothe) to provide some flavor of their insights into the significance of their work. The quotations are anonymous to preserve confidentiality. (Readers who are interested in an area of research cited should see Appendix A: Awardees of the Research Development Program and Their Areas of Study as of March 1, 1973.) Perhaps the quotations will also communicate some of the enthusiasm common to many investigators, despite the rigors and frustrations of pursuing "hard truth."

In the discussion that follows, the topics of interest have been divided into five major areas—psychiatric treatment, psychopathology, psychopharmacology, social and biological bases of behavior, and child development—and one minor area, unclassified. Table 1 gives a statistical summary of the number of program participants working in each area, although a given investigator's work may fall into several classifications; note areas of secondary concentration in Table 1. Furthermore, there is extensive cross-fertilization, both methodologically and substantively, across disciplinary and topical boundaries. The five major research areas have thus been analytically separated only for the sake of discussion; the fact of their increasing convergence represents a major step toward understanding and treating the whole man.

## Psychiatric Treatment

From the perspective of the psychiatric clinician, the entire behavioral science emerging from psychiatric research has important implications for improved psychiatric treatment. The causes of psychiatric disorders (social, psychological, and physiological), their underlying base and developmental preconditions, as well as the psychopharmacological effects of drugs are all research areas in which expanded knowledge can contribute ultimately to better treatment. Thus there is no clear line between research of practical application to daily clinical work and that which may have a more indirect influence by its effect on theory or diagnostic procedure.

The range of studies conducted by program participants that are related, directly or indirectly, to psychiatric treatment includes investigations of long-recognized problems and familiar treatment methods as well as studies of new experimental approaches to treatment.

Among the individual programs of research supported by the Research Development Program, studies of the doctor-patient relationship and its effects on particular symptoms or symptom complexes are among

Table 1. Research Areas of Primary and Secondary Concentration of 169 Participants in NIMH Research Development Program

| Research Area | Number of Scientists | | |
|---|---|---|---|
| | Primary Research Area | Secondary Research Area* | Total |
| Psychiatric treatment | 14 | 6 | 20 |
| Psychopathology | | | |
|   General | 17 ⎫ | 17 ⎫ | 34 ⎫ |
|   Schizophrenia | 7 ⎬ 40 | 4 ⎬ 27 | 11 ⎬ 67 |
|   Depression | 4 | 2 | 6 |
|   Psychosomatic | 12 ⎭ | 4 ⎭ | 16 ⎭ |
| Psychopharmacology | 14 | 9 | 23 |
| Social and biological | | | |
|   bases of behavior | | | |
|   Biochemistry | 15 ⎫ | 0 ⎫ | 15 ⎫ |
|   Neurophysiology | 26 ⎬ 62 | 1 ⎬ 6 | 27 ⎬ 68 |
|   Sleep and dreaming | 10 | 4 | 14 |
|   Personality development | 11 ⎭ | 1 ⎭ | 12 ⎭ |
| Child development | 36 | 7 | 43 |
| Unclassified (creativity | | | |
|   and history of psychiatry) | 3 | 0 | 3 |
| Total | 169 | 55 | 224 |

* Of the 169 participants, 55 were classified again by area of secondary concentration.

the most directly relevant to improving treatment techniques. These programs are primarily conducted to determine and quantify relationships among factors in psychotherapy or to test whether reliable methods of treatment can be designed to relieve particular symptoms. Studies deal with aspects of nonverbal and verbal communication in the psychiatric interview; the therapist's interventions, attitudes, and concepts; the accuracy of his judgment about "bad" and "good" sessions; and his observation of symptom formation in his patient.

Several long-term investigations of psychoanalytic treatment have been undertaken. Given the extensiveness of the data to be analyzed and the technical and professional difficulties of recording and coding them, a degree of determination and resourcefulness unusual even for a scientist is required. Nonetheless, one investigator is developing quantitative scales of verbal behavior that will permit the content of analytical sessions to be measured and described in terms of specific amounts of anxiety, hostility, social alienation, and personal disorganization. In another approach to treatment, verbal interactions of patient and therapist are being studied to validate psychoanalytic conclusions and to disentangle substantive issues in psychiatric treatment from the effects of the interpersonal relationship. In a related study, computer content analysis is used to describe the frequency and patterning of words and concepts in the course of psychoanalytic treatment. The investigator conducting this study has described his overall goals as follows:

> I am trying to put the study of what happens during a psychoanalytic process on a truly scientific basis by developing ways to measure objectively the many variables that analysts and psychotherapists have thought to be important in understanding the motivations and personalities of persons undergoing psychoanalysis. The most promising of these methods is that of computer content-analysis. Every session of a psychoanalysis is tape recorded. Computer programs look up each word of the complete, transcribed text, assign the words to conceptual categories and keep track of the frequency of each concept in each session. These concepts (considered variables) may then be clustered (by factor-analysis and other procedures) and the frequencies graphed over time to give a quantitative description of the course of the analysis.
>
> Using these and similar methods, I have been able to plot the course of an analysis that became stalemated and in which the patient did not improve. An independent summary of the analysis dramatically corresponds to the course revealed by the plots. Thus, for example, one can show quite rigorously the fact and nature of the changes in what the patient talked about and how she talked on such occasions as when the analyst left to have a baby, or when the patient began an affair, had an abortion, or relived jealous rage at the birth of a sister.
>
> My major plans include helping to establish a large library of completely tape-recorded psychoanalyses (to serve as a basic source of documents for numerous future studies) and to continue development of a psychoanalytic computer dictionary. I will also continue to record a case that I am now analyzing. . . .
>
> Psychoanalysis has long been regarded as a basic clinical method for extensive, detailed study of motivation and personality in mentally ill people. Unfortunately, the scientific study of the psychoanalytic process has not kept pace with the pervasive influence of psychoanalytic theoretical concepts in the humanities, psychology, and psychiatry. My work is designed to help redeem the promise of psychoanalysis as a science.

Statistical techniques such as those being used in this study are also being applied to the study of practitioners' motivations and personalities in psychoanalysis.

In methodology and content, several studies of therapeutic conditioning techniques are similar. For the most part, a given behavioral problem is viewed as a response to stress. It may be treated either as an entity in itself or as an essential aspect of some major illness such as schizophrenia. Therapy is based on the observation that stress in interpersonal relations produces tension (manifested by such symptoms as defensive and hostile feelings, anxiety, stuttering, frigidity in sexual relations, muscular tightness or spasticity, headache, sweating palms, increased heart rate, or higher blood pressure). The stress can be relieved or controlled as patients learn relaxation techniques with the aid of instrumentation that monitors and provides electronic feedback of their responses. As described by one investigator using this technique:

> Our major aim is to teach people greater voluntary control over their own physiological responses by means of electronic information feedback techniques. . . .
> We plan to continue what has become the central emphasis of the research in our laboratory—modification of the individual's maladaptive response to stress. A good deal of our current work lies in the area of behavior therapy—using relaxation as a means of desensitizing patients to specific anxieties such as examination anxiety, public speaking anxiety, and so forth. Exploratory work is also being conducted in using the relaxation technique in cases of difficult-to-treat pervasive or "free-floating" anxiety. A major component of pervasive anxiety disorders is the patients' very high levels of physiological arousal. We think that systematic relaxation training would be helpful in teaching these patients to lower their arousal levels and to lower the high anxiety associated with these high levels of arousal.
> We believe the feedback training techniques have potential application to a variety of psychosomatic stress-related disorders. A major component of these disorders is an acquired over-reaction to stress. In many patients, even imagining a feared situation will provoke a vigorous stress reaction. In our work to date with tension headache, a stress-related psychosomatic disorder, our results have been most encouraging.
> Perhaps feedback techniques can be used to teach people control over various maladaptive stress reactions involved in a great many psychosomatic disorders. Eventually, psychosomatic patients may learn to lower [their] blood pressure, reduce [their] heart rate or gastric motility, and other visceral responses by means of feedback training techniques. Recent work, such as that of Neal Miller, demonstrates that visceral learning can be accomplished in animals. Similar training may be possible in humans. Such training could have extensive application to the vast domain of human psychosomatic disease—an area of medicine in which progress has been relatively modest.

A promising extension of behavior therapy by yet another investigator consists of using videotape feedback for treating patients with character disorders, such as criminals and juvenile delinquents. In another study, tools are being developed to aid in visceral learning; as indicated in the quotation above, this technique may later be used extensively for treatment of psychosomatic disorders.

*Psychopathology*

*General Problems of Psychopathology.* The nature of adult psychopathology, both physiological and behavioral, presents a natural area for study by the research-oriented psychiatrist. In the psychopathology studies supported by the Research Development Program, research directed primarily to behavioral and physiological symptoms, rather than to the etiology or effects of a specific disease, has been predominant. Of the scientists conducting research in psychopathology, over half have been studying broad psychopathology problems that they have labeled *affective disorders, psychoses, affective psychoses,* or just *psychiatric disorders.*

Psychiatric patients are generally studied to identify neurological and biochemical correlates of their psychopathological behavior, such as enzyme abnormalities or deviant patterns seen in evoked cerebral electrophysiological responses. Some studies focus on the effect of central nervous system-active drugs on chemical agents in synaptic transmission or on neurophysiological aspects of sensory and cardiovascular functioning among schizophrenic, aged, and brain-damaged patients. Research into brain abnormalities underlying clinical problems such as epilepsy and violent behavior is conducted by one investigator using stereotactic electrode implantation on animals (a technique whereby very precise three-dimensional localization of brain sites is possible). Another investigator, working with a group of colleagues, has directed a research ward of severely ill patients. Among the problems studied has been cognitive impairment from electroshock.

Symptoms of disturbed cognitive behavior in mental illness—such as intrusive thought (lack of control of one's thinking) and the distortion of time sense—have occupied two investigators who have studied these phenomena in psychotics, depressives, and drug users. They are experimenting with treatment procedures for specific symptom relief. One describes his studies as follows:

> An extensive sense of time is a distinctive human characteristic that enables man to cope with anticipated environmental and personal changes through bringing the future into the psychological present. Different belief systems emerge according to how man

construes his future; these expectations guide his current action. Some individuals, however, become alienated from society because they misconstrue their future. A paranoid person, for example, becomes gripped by a fixed expectation that he attempts to validate by garnering remembrances, rather than testing his hunches in the future. We have evidence that psychotic disorganization, which includes the dissolution of the self and the emergence of irrational thought, stems from a confusion of the past, present, and future. This is true for clinical acute psychoses as well as psychoses induced by . . . drugs such as marijuana. We have also shown how temporal distortions are related to depression, delinquency, suicide attempts, and acts of violence. Much of our work has focused on how the distorted appraisal of outcomes gives rise to emotions that have gone awry and that thereby serve as spurs to aberrant acts.

Research on psychopathology also extends to a related study in which distorted belief systems, as in paranoia, are explored by computer techniques and contrasted with normal belief systems.

Sexual phenomena in psychopathology have been investigated from a variety of approaches: extensive and intensive, biochemical, social, and psychological. These studies are concerned with problems as varied as the relationship of sex hormones and adrenocortical steroids to depression and aggression, hormonal abnormality and gender dimorphic behavior, sexual problems related to pregnancy and contraception, the social effects of obscenity and pornography, and the relationship of male and female homosexuality to psychiatric disorders. In one interdisciplinary study of sexual psychopathology, an investigator conducts animal studies on the effects of hormonal imbalance, behavioral studies of boys with cross-gender behavior, and family studies and psychoanalytic investigations of male trans-sexuals and mothers of boys with cross-gender behavior.

Several aspects of alcoholism have come under study by a number of psychiatric researchers. Both the metabolic and behavioral aspects of alcoholism are being explored by one investigator who for a number of years has directed a large laboratory. Another investigator of alcoholism combines studies of environmental and genetic factors in the etiology of alcoholism with a study of the effects of alcoholism on memory and learning. In yet another line of alcoholism research, a biochemist primarily interested in the behavioral function of enzymes is studying the effect of ethanol on brain-protein synthesis. A behavioral study of the way alcoholic fathers affect their families has demonstrated a pathological effect on their daughters.

Epidemiological and cultural or social studies are vigorously represented in research on psychopathology. Among the socially oriented scientists, cultural, social, and economic factors in psychiatric illness have been investigated. In one study, a group of superior college sophomores, on whom extensive longitudinal data had been collected, is compared with delinquents and deprived urban non-delinquents to reveal factors in successful adaptation, alcoholism, drug abuse, and mental illness. In a related line of study, an urban sociologist analyzes life histories of both deprived and middle-class blacks to determine childhood factors that predict occupational success, criminal behavior, and psychiatric disorder. To make possible effective guidelines for mental health programs among minority groups, particularly Indians, another social scientist has been studying psychiatric illness in relation to cultural, ecological, and familial factors among Hopis and Navajos. Yet another investigator has extended his research on the relation between social status and psychiatric disorder to five ethnic groups—white Anglo-Saxon Protestants, Jews, Irish, blacks, and Puerto Ricans—distinguishing between the advantaged and the disadvantaged in each group. Other investigators have tried to improve theory and classification of psychiatric disorders.

*Schizophrenia.*    Among the specific psychopathological problems receiving considerable research attention is schizophrenia, including its biochemistry, its origin in the family environment, its psychological deficits, its physiological symptoms, and its response to certain forms of treatment.

One investigator has aided understanding of the etiology and phenomenology of schizophrenia through long-term family studies. He has compared upper-middle-class families having delinquent offspring, families with schizophrenic members, and normal families. Another extension of family study and research on schizophrenia focuses on family structure and style and the role of the schizophrenic child. This investigator has summarized his work and suggested future directions for schizophrenia research:

> I believe that my work over the past 15 years, particularly concerning the etiology of schizophrenia, has had a very significant impact on both the treatment of schizophrenia and research concerning its etiology. Numerous investigators have followed the lead of studying the families of schizophrenic patients. The work has also raised challenges to more purely genetic concepts of the etiology of schizophrenia, which has led to re-evaluation of the earlier genetic studies. . . .
>
> Concerning future work, I believe there is a great need to re-examine schizophrenic syndromes because the clinical pictures have changed markedly with changes in hospital care and the use of tranquilizers, but such changes have not been clearly defined. I think it essential to gain clearer insights into just what changes in the patients' thought processes, emotional control, and in other

areas during remissions in order to better understand the therapeutic process, including the effect of tranquilizers on schizophrenic
patients. There is also a need to examine the relationships between
psychoses precipitated by LSD and related drugs to schizophrenic
disorganizations and to sort out the overlap and differences.

Patients with schizophrenic reactions still remain the largest
group of patients in mental hospitals; I believe our investigations
have helped clarify something of the etiology and have helped produce new methods of treatment involving the patient's family.

During the past several years, through collaborative studies with
mental hospitals under the auspices of the psychopharmacology research
program of the NIMH, the effects of antipsychotic drugs (the phenothiazines) have been tested as a means of establishing and maintaining the
emotional stability of schizophrenic patients. These studies have shown
that environmental factors in the patients' life histories conditioned the
effectiveness of the various antipsychotic drugs.

In another line of psychopharmacological schizophrenia research,
a behavioral scientist has designed a study to test the effects of antipsychotic drugs on psychological process in schizophrenic patients. He
administers psychological tests at appropriate times in the course of drug
treatment (at the outset, after sustained medication, and on withdrawal
of the drugs) and measures specific cognitive capacities—for example, for
retention, abstract thinking, and attention.

Other schizophrenia studies are directed to the way psychological
deficits in schizophrenia are related to biochemical and neurophysiological
deficits. Still others focus on particular symptoms in schizophrenia and
psychophysiological relationships: the abnormal methylation of dopamine
in schizophrenia; the cortical responses of schizophrenic patients correlated
with early life experiences; cortical evoked potentials correlated with behavioral variability among schizophrenic patients; and abnormalities in the
EEG recordings of those who are outstandingly poor on attention tests
and correspondingly unresponsive to phenothiazines. The latter study has
been described by the primary investigator as follows:

> The major objective of our research is (a) to explore the nature
> and role of disordered attention in schizophrenic patients, and
> (b) to develop relevant animal models that will permit pharma-
> cological manipulation and testing of hypotheses concerning the
> underlying neural variables. . . .
>
> We have been able to divide chronic schizophrenic patients into
> two groups based on their performance on a simple test of atten-
> tion. The two groups do not differ in ability to perform on simple
> cognitive tests, nor do they differ in sub-types of schizophrenia,
> length of hospitalization, age of onset of disease, or in other ways.

The only significant predictor of poor performance on the attention test is a history of mental illness in the family and, more specifically, a mentally ill sibling. We are at present engaged in experiments designed to test the hypothesis that these patients with poor performance are in a state of chronic central arousal. We are doing this by comparing their response to various drugs and looking for differences in their EEG. Data obtained thus far suggest that the poor performers as compared to good performers have less alpha [waves] on the EEG, are less responsive to single doses of phenothiazine drugs, but not barbiturates, and have difficulty maintaining a readiness to respond in reaction-time experiments. . . .

The work on schizophrenia has special relevance to the understanding of the disease. At a simple applied level, our data suggest that we may be able to identify those schizophrenic patients most likely to respond in a positive way to phenothiazine medication.

At a more basic level, an understanding of the role of the arousal system in schizophrenia may allow us to determine effective measures of interrupting the disease or even possibly preventing it.

Other research is exploring the finding that the effects on animal behavior of compounds found in the urine of schizophrenic patients resemble those of drugs such as LSD. A more behavioral study of schizophrenia is based on the observation that schizophrenic patients suffer from an overarousal characteristic of strong negative emotion, which in turn produces skeletal muscle tension. One investigator is using behavior therapy to test the psychophysiological relationship: can psychological symptoms be reduced when muscle tension is lessened? He has projected the potential benefits of his study:

If methods of this kind should prove therapeutically effective, they would have some practical advantages. For example, current drug therapies for schizophrenia have a number of associated side effects, but it is difficult to imagine undesirable side effects resulting from voluntary use of skeletal muscle relaxation. Second, training in muscle relaxation using our methods can be conducted by a minimally trained person. A single professional probably could supervise the work of a number of such people, whereas traditional psychotherapy is generally thought to require large amounts of professional time and is probably ineffective with schizophrenics.

*Depressive Disorders.*   Research on depression is directed primarily to biological, biochemical, and hormonal disturbances in the depressive state as well as to its psychological accompaniments. Many of the investigators conducting these studies test the effectiveness of drugs on physiological and emotional symptoms.

Imbalance in hormone systems is often associated with severe depressive and manic illness. For example, endocrine disturbance is associated with precise clinical features of the depressive illness and all the hormones affected in depression are regulated by the hypothalamus. The goal of research by one investigator, therefore, is to identify the physiological and biochemical imbalances occurring in the depressive state and to understand how treatment with lithium carbonate (a promising preventive of depressive behavior) affects physical symptoms.

Other experiments on psychopharmacology in depression test the therapeutic effectiveness of thyroid hormone in combination with other drugs:

> My work is directed toward illuminating the role of biological factors in the cause, perpetuation, relapse, and treatment of the affective disorders, particularly depression. Most of the knowledge in this area has derived from treatment. For example, by knowing that imipramine usually relieves depression and that reserpine sometimes produces it, and by studying the cellular action of these drugs, we have gained insight into the biochemical conditions that may obtain in the brains of depressed patients. I have therefore adopted the strategy of finding and then studying substances that produce a clinical difference.
>
> Proceeding from clinical observations, my colleagues and I have shown in a series of double blind, placebo-controlled studies that depressed patients, when treated with imipramine, recover twice as fast if they are given at the same time either a small dose of triiodothyronine or two injections of thyroid-stimulating hormone. Thus the morbidity of the condition is reduced by half, as is the danger of mortality through suicide. Our studies have been replicated by two other groups. Neither they nor we have noted increased toxicity from the experimental treatments. . . .
>
> This work is very relevant to the problem of mental health. In Western civilization, one man in 100 and two women in 100 will be hospitalized at least once for depression. Many others will be treated as outpatients and still others will go undetected. This enormous prevalence of depression contributes substantially to the high incidence of suicide. A safe, rapid, effective treatment will surely contribute to the effective management of the problem. When the mechanism of this treatment is fully understood, it will be applied to the greater task of prevention.

In female outpatients with depressive disorders, changes in metabolism of specific brain chemicals (catecholamines) in response to drug treatment are also under study. The author of a widely known depression scale is concentrating on sleep disturbance in depression.

In laboratory studies, depressive syndromes are created in animal subjects to observe the origin of depression and the effects of various types of therapy. An investigator working with pigtail, bonnet macaque, and squirrel monkeys has created a promising animal model of human depression:

> My research is concerned with the impact of the mother-infant relationship on infant social development; in particular, the development of infant attachments is viewed as the major dimension to be studied by means of both experimental and normative developmental approaches. Since the work is carried out with non-human primates but gains its major conceptual impetus from child development research, a strong comparative emphasis is maintained in which several species are utilized to enhance the likelihood of producing results of broad evolutionary significance. At present, three species—the pigtail, the bonnet macaque, and the squirrel monkey—are under intensive study. . . .
>
> As a continuation of previous studies on separation from the mother, we have completed an assessment of the changing responses to mother during a prolonged separation period in both pigtails and bonnets. This study indicates that a dramatic, *reproducible* depression can be evoked in separated pigtail infants by presenting them with the lost mother figure. Bonnet infants under the same circumstances, while failing to show depressive responses, show an enhancement of their adoptive relationship with other adults in the group when their own mother is returned briefly during the separation interval. . . .
>
> The implications of this research in the mental health area relate to the importance of attachments for normal behavioral growth in children, the significance of maternal loss in humans, and the widespread appearance of depression as a basic psychopathological state. By maintaining a broad comparative perspective, it is hoped that some appreciation of evolutionary continuity in these significant areas may be generated and thus provide meaningful hypotheses to be tested further at the human level. The depression generated in our separated pigtail infants, for example, in terms of origin and overt manifestation, more closely resembles the depression frequently seen in children and adults than any other form previously described in the experimental animal literature. The variables that seem to influence the development of infant attachment and the consequent response to maternal loss in monkeys suggests that we may be able to assess the impact of disruptions and disturbances in early attachment processes (such as may occur to children of broken homes) and the means of alleviating their long-term effects; we may also gain an understanding of factors that may operate during traumatic though temporary loss of attachment figures, as may occur during hospitalization or as a consequence of removal of the infant or parent from the home for varying periods.

*Psychosomatic Disorders.*    Psychosomatic research, either into the relation between the physical and psychological aspects of specific psychosomatic diseases or in disease processes in general, occupies the majority of researchers in this survey who have been studying specific psychopathological problems.

There is sufficient evidence from their work, taken collectively, to demonstrate that the past 20 years have seen significant theoretical change as well as considerable expansion and increasing complexity of the phenomena studied in psychosomatic research. Previously, only diseases in a fairly limited range of gastrointestinal, asthmatic, and arthritic disorders were considered to be of definitely psychic origin. In current research, however, the emphasis is not so much on psychic origin and treatment by psychotherapy as it is on the complex interplay of physiological and emotional factors in a considerably broader range of diseases.

Thus, one investigator, who formerly studied emotional correlates of gastrointestinal disease, is now engaged with problems in patients' adaptation to a blood disease treatment: maintenance hemodialysis. Another investigator and his co-workers have long been concerned with the role of psychological factors in the course and onset of illness, irrespective of diagnosis. Recently they have been studying psychophysiological phenomena in a variety of traumatic experiences: sudden death, stroke, and multiple sclerosis:

> This research has been concerned primarily with an attempt to achieve a better understanding of the relationship between mental or emotional health and physical disease. It has involved studying the life setting in which illness develops and has demonstrated that both physical and mental disease may ensue when the individual feels unable to cope and gives up.
>
> Currently we are concerned with investigation of these relationships in particular groups of patients—namely, sudden death, stroke, and multiple sclerosis. At the same time in experimental situations, we are studying endocrine and other physiological changes associated with the affects of giving up. Other investigations are concerned with the psychological mechanisms and social factors that are conducive to the maintenance of health. Others working in the research program are exploring the application of these findings to the improvement of the care of the sick, especially those with life-threatening conditions where unfavorable emotional reactions may tip the balance toward a bad outcome—patients undergoing renal hemodialysis, permanent implantation of pacemakers, renal transplantation, cardiac catheterization, or open-heart surgery. . . . or those in coronary care units. . . .
>
> Probably the most important implication of this work in relationship to problems of mental health is the demonstration that the psychological well-being of the individual is vital for his physical as well as mental health. This indicates a fundamental unity between mental and physical health and emphasizes the great im-

portance and potential contribution to mental health of the general physician who recognizes these inter-relationships and is properly trained to help. The research has had a major impact on the educational program at this university and has important implications for the development of patterns of medical care.

Even in more traditional areas of psychosomatic research, such as asthma, the perspective has broadened. As studies of bronchial asthma have progressed, methods for the quantitative assessment of data on psychic history and conflict (as provided by psychoanalytic interviews) have been developed, and both animal experiments and methods for physiological measurement with human subjects have been used. Physiological indices developed in a laboratory study have been applied by one investigator to speech production and the respiratory cycle of asthmatic patients. Another investigator is comparing psychological factors in the precipitation and development of human asthma cases with the effect of such influences as stress from separation or isolation on bronchial asthma in animals.

Other investigators, taking a broad view of psychosomatic diseases, explore the relations among stress, blood viscosity, and circulatory disease and the psychological components of heart disease, skin disorder, and rheumatoid arthritis. Psychological disorders in relation to physical disturbance in obesity and epilepsy are also under study. The range of behavior of epileptics being studied includes behavioral correlates of limbic and cortical functions and the diurnal and nocturnal cycles of electrophysiological and behavioral phenomena.

One investigator (who has frequently written on progress in psychosomatic medicine) has conducted experiments that have extended variously to the perceptual and cardiovascular responses of ulcer patients, the psychophysiological aspects of cardiovascular disease, and psychoendocrine considerations in breast cancer.

Among the laboratory studies being conducted, one team of investigators is concerned mainly with psychosomatic phenomena in the pre- and postnatal development of animal subjects. Their experiments are designed to clarify how environmental deprivation affects susceptibility to diseases and to measure adrenal medullary and adrenocortical activity as functions of psychological manipulation.

Techniques and objectives of psychosomatic research are frequently shared by scientists in other areas of psychiatric research. Given the fluid interchange among research areas, it is not unusual for a behavior therapist, for example, to contribute to the understanding of psychosomatic relationships through his study of relaxation techniques for physical symptoms of phobia.

*Psychopharmacology.* In psychiatric research, psychopharmacology occupies a strategically central position. Although its historical background is recent (only in the past 15 to 20 years has treatment by psychotropic drugs become a significant practice in mental hospitals), this area of study is of extreme interest both to mental health professionals and to the public at large. It is widely appreciated that the whole prospect of psychiatric treatment has been changed dramatically by psychotropic drugs and that the whole community mental health movement would have been virtually impossible without them.

This section will examine the work of scientists who are concentrating on the problems of psychopharmacological drug use and abuse. At present, since more is known of the behavioral and clinical effects of these drugs than of their underlying physiological mechanisms, most of these scientists are working to clarify the physiology of drug response. Their studies are trying to define the precise relations between physiological mechanisms and behavioral effects on mood, attitude, perception, attention, and memory as well as to identify the social factors that affect both drug use and response.

Among the physiologically oriented studies being conducted, one representative and productive investigator is working to clarify the function of naturally occurring amines (catecholamines, serotonin, histamine) as transmitters in the nervous system; he is also working to clarify their interactions with drugs. The question of how different types of neurons respond to such drugs as amphetamines is also under investigation. Experimental models are being developed that may aid in predicting drug effects on individuals with specific diseases. For example, one scientist is studying the effect of amphetamines on hyperactivity. In another study, data are being obtained on cerebral evoked responses to specific drugs in patients, normals, and animal subjects. Alterations in various parts of the human central nervous system are recorded; such changes can then be localized experimentally through animal studies.

The effects of LSD and related drugs on the metabolism of serotonin and subsequent changes in cellular enzymatic manipulation provide keys to understanding drug effects as well as the function of amines in transmitting impulses through the nervous system. A psychologist with extensive training in biochemistry combines approaches from different areas of research to explore both catecholamine effects on various aspects of behavior (as manipulated by drugs), and the effects of various types of (operant conditioning) training on catecholamine levels. The confirmed data are used to elucidate a complex relationship for which a single technical approach would be inadequate.

Special studies by other investigators focus on psychological factors that affect reactions to psychotropic drugs. Investigators are also exploring the effects of drugs on learning and attention, on maladaptive behavior, on school phobias, and on hyperactivity in children.

Among the basic studies that are essential for understanding psychopharmacology is one in which a biochemist is investigating the effects of drugs on biochemical and central nervous system development at organismic and cellular levels.

At a more clinical level, several studies are directed at psychological and sociological factors in drug use and abuse. For example, a sociologist is studying the effect of drugs (therapeutic or psychotogenic) on family behavior. Research by a psychopharmacologist on drug abuse and the psychopathology of drug use is directed to the effects of chronic use of LSD or marijuana on mental functions and psychological behavior, as well as to social phenomena that either lead to or result from the use of psychotogenic drugs.

Using animal subjects, another investigator is studying both the reward potential of drugs that act as psychomotor stimulators and the conditions of deprivation that affect addiction. Research is also designed to clarify the neurophysiological effects of LSD, marijuana, and alcohol and the relevance of such data to social problems. One investigator who is exploring hallucinogenic drug effects has summarized the relationship between laboratory studies and ultimate clinical benefits that may result:

> The problems of our research are (1) to analyze the behavioral effects of hallucinogenic or psychotomimetic drugs, such as LSD, and (2) to determine the role of certain endogenous monoamines, such as serotonin (5-HT) and norepinephrine (NE), in some of these effects. . . .
>
> The importance to psychiatry and mental health of understanding the effects of hallucinogenic or psychotomimetic drugs is obvious. There is clearly a growing drug problem in certain important segments of contemporary society that cannot be solved until we understand both the state the drug induces and why such a state can be reinforcing. Our research is relevant to drug abuse and treatment in that it is directly concerned with the supposedly unique properties of these compounds and the reason often given for their self-administration: their ability to alter reality. But do the drugs in fact change the way we hear, see, and so on (our reality)—that is, do they alter sensitivity or do they modify some other aspect of how we normally respond, perhaps changing our motivation or our desire for various objects? The development of effective treatment would seem to await the answer to this question. It is one thing to try to reestablish the individual's motivation, interest in life, or even respect for contemporary values but quite another to try to restore normal perceptual processes.

It has become clear that hallucinogenic drugs often affect sub-human animals in analogous ways. Therefore, further studies of animals will not only help elucidate the mechanisms underlying perceptual behavior but also will be relevant to drug-behavior inter-actions in humans. Once we clearly understand how the complex but well controlled behavior being studied in our experiments is affected by the drugs, appropriate studies involving human subjects can be designed. In any case, animals will continue to be used in the search for neural and biochemical correlates of drug effect, the knowledge of which is mandatory for pharmacological treatment of "bad trips."

Both acute drug effects and the phenomenon of drug tolerance require greater research to aid in the treatment of drug addiction. In one study designed to improve the therapy of addicts, clinical research in psychopharmacology extends to the operation of a large treatment center where different treatment programs may be compared.

Much of this research suggests the importance of distinguishing between psychopharmacological and other factors as they influence psychiatric treatment. Clarifying this issue is the special province of yet another psychiatric researcher, who is developing computer techniques for multi-factorial analysis of clinical psychopharmacological data.

The impact of psychopharmacological research is far more widespread than delineating drug effects. For example, in basic studies of human behavior by neuroscientists, techniques derived from psychopharmacology have contributed much to the efficiency and flexibility of the research.

### Social and Biological Bases of Behavior

By far the greatest area of concentration in psychiatric research supported by the Research Development Program concerns the social and biological bases of behavior. While the objective of this research is to clarify mechanisms, developmental sequences, or functions in behavior rather than to study some aspect of psychopathology or treatment, the impact of the clinical setting is nonetheless evident in all parts of the research, and a majority of the scientists give specific attention to problems related to psychopathology.

We will discuss here four major topics of interest to the scientists conducting basic studies: the biochemical bases of behavior, the neurophysiological bases of behavior, sleep and dreaming, and personality development and social and environmental adaptation.

*The Biochemical Bases of Behavior.*   Research into the biochemistry of behavior is closely related to both neurophysiological and psychopharmacological studies; indeed, these areas often overlap. The biochemical research sponsored by the Research Development Program primarily investigates the chemical substrate of the nervous system and relates chemical reactions to their behavioral consequences.

Key foci of research include the distribution and levels of biochemical substances in the brain and the relationship between the functions of the endocrine system and the central nervous system. For example, specific studies are directed to the brain mechanisms that control corticosteroids and the adrenal steroids (which are used as therapeutic agents for cerebral-vascular accidents and multiple sclerosis).

A crucial question that is frequently asked is, "how are biogenic amines such as epinephrine and serotonin synthesized?" Since the operation of the amines affects synaptic transmission and therefore neural activity, the amines are an important focus of much of the research. One investigator summarized the significance of such studies:

> We are conducting research on the biochemical physiology of central synaptic transmission and the way it is affected by drugs. The work's importance seems to lie in its contributions to understanding basic biochemical and metabolic mechanisms controlling the activity of chemically mediated synapses in the central nervous system. That understanding can help clarify mechanisms of action of centrally active drugs, including tranquilizers, antidepressants, lithium salts used in mania, and drugs such as DOPA and Amantadine, used in Parkinsonism. Finally, the work is relevant to an understanding of biochemical abnormalities that have profound neuropsychiatric consequences in hepatic failure and Parkinsonism, probably in affective psychoses, and possibly in schizophrenia. Amine-mediated central transmission can be claimed to be our best present active lead in attempting to understand possible biological bases of several psychoses and the mechanisms of action of most of the drugs found to be effective in psychiatric illness.

The psychopharmacological chain is gradually becoming clearer. Drug intervention affects amine biosynthesis, and so, by modifying synaptic transmission, has behavioral consequences. In addition, the use of drugs as a research tool can illuminate the basic biochemical and metabolic mechanisms that control the activity of chemically mediated synapses in the central nervous system. Hence, students of these mechanisms make use of centrally active drugs, including tranquilizers and antidepressants, in this manner.

This research is applicable to various disorders, including alcoholism, Parkinsonism, and affective psychoses. For example, understanding the effects of ethanol on brain-protein synthesis may lead to biochemical treatment and/or prevention of alcoholism. Much of the research in Parkinsonism and in the affective psychoses is devoted to the role of biogenic amines in certain brain dysfunctions.

The biochemical approach is also used to clarify the whole mechanism—chemical, neuronal, and behavioral—of aggression. As a key to the causes of aggressive behavior, adrenal hormones, sex hormones, and the neuroendocrine processes are studied with reference to the sites and mechanisms of sexual differentiation in the mammalian brain. Hormone injections during the neonatal period are known to affect various central nervous system functions that can (via the neuroendocrine system) lead to abnormal androgen metabolism in adolescence. This, in turn, can be a physiological correlate of violent behavior. One avenue of research is therefore concerned with the balance of hormonal activity in male or female functional development and with how hormonal imbalance may lead to sexual malfunctioning or aggression.

Neurochemical changes also accompany the effects of severe stress. Such changes in the metabolism of hormones can be studied in animals subjected to physical and emotional stress; drugs to reverse these changes are also tested in stressed animal subjects.

As shown in the preceding discussion, study of the biochemical correlates of emotional and other psychiatric disorders is also clearly an integral part of the research in psychopathology and psychopharmacology. As will be seen, it is integral to child development research as well.

*The Neurophysiological Bases of Behavior.* Questions concerning the neurophysiological roots of behavior pervade the whole spectrum of psychiatric investigation; ultimately, knowledge of mind rests on comprehending the brain that underlies it. Yet answers to neurophysiological questions are painfully hard to come by. They originate in such an awesome complex of microbiological relationships, require such advanced technical skills, and demand investigations at levels of such relative simplicity and specificity that clinically relevant data often seem elusive. Nonetheless, since the importance of the problems outweighs the difficulty of solving them, a large component of psychiatric research is devoted to understanding the physical foundations of the psyche.

The specialized experimental research in neurophysiological processes conducted by program participants focuses on a multitude of mechanisms in the central and autonomic nervous systems. It is concerned with all pathways in the reception of sensory stimuli (with emphasis on auditory and visual), and with information processing from the spinal cord through the brain stem and cerebellum and into the cortex.

Individual investigations usually concentrate on special functions of certain areas, such as those of the hippocampus and the thalamus. Electrical activity of the central nervous system is charted, from the operation of a single neuron to the mechanisms of strategic centers in behavioral functioning. Studies of brain development encompass both ontogenetic and phylogenetic investigations and comparisons.

Techniques that have been refined for neurophysiological research extend from microbiological analysis and recordings from microelectrodes to electrical stimulation of the brain and surgical ablation. Other investigations into neurophysiological functioning may involve stress or excitement, nutritional or other deprivation in the neonate animal, or pharmacological manipulation. The technique of the cold probe is also available, by which a thermal dysfunction of an area of the central nervous system may be used as an experimental condition. An investigator using this technique, among others, has presented the results and rationale of his study as follows:

My research is directed toward elucidating some of the fundamental principles of function of the human brain. I am particularly interested in the neurophysiological mechanisms that constitute the functional substrate of perception and emotion. Most of the work being done by me and my collaborators is conducted in the laboratory using subhuman primates.

It has been established by us that the perception of sensory events is controlled and regulated to a significant extent by the activity of cellular pools in certain structures of the brain stem. We have found also that some chemical substances, such as LSD and amphetamine, which modify the electrical activity of nerve cells in these structures, have definite effects on sensory information processing. As a continuation of this work, we are currently investigating the cerebral mechanisms at the basis of perceptual attention and short-term memory. In this study we are using the method of direct nerve-cell recording during behavioral tests. Selective functional inactivation of parts of the brain by application of cold with special implanted thermoelectric probes is another of the methods used. These methods have been developed in my laboratory and are suited for use in the awake, free-moving animal. We have found that the cryogenic block of the cerebral cortex of the frontal lobe produces a reversible deficit of short-term memory function. This finding is now being further investigated and followed by study of nerve-cell activity during transient memory tests, both in normal conditions and during frontal lobe cooling. In addition, we are exploring the cerebral processes of information handling in signal detection tasks, with the aim of finding out which are the critical behavioral and electro-physiological variables affecting the perception of environmental events by the organism. The significance of this research for clinical psychiatry is clear because disorders of attention occupy a cardinal position in the psychopathology of a number of deranged mental conditions such as manic-depressive psychosis, obsessive-compulsive neurosis, infantile autism, and toxic psychoses. Pursuing a special interest in the latter group of disorders, we plan to investigate in detail the effects of alcohol on information transmission in the brain. We then hope to be able to unravel some of the pharmacodynamic effects of alcohol on brain function.

A scientific understanding of neurophysiological research would require considerable background in the history, status, and methodology of the neuro-sciences. Perhaps a brief review of the problems, stated in behavioral terms, with which neurophysiologists in psychiatric research are engaged will clarify this area.

Advanced studies of neurotransmission in the brain are directed to fundamental processes at the level of individual cells; to the interaction of neurons with surrounding interstitial fluid, with glia, and with other neurons through synapses; and to the response of tissues to changes in chemistry, morphology, metabolism, and electrophysiological characteristics. This is the kind of work on which biochemical, pharmacological, physiological, and psychological understanding of mental functions will ultimately depend.

By studying synaptic physiology in a relatively simple organism, an investigator can trace complex behavioral sequences from their initiation in single neurons and can relate specific behavioral consequences to individual identifiable neurons. In a simple organism, alterations in the efficacy of synaptic connections are demonstrated to effect habituation and dishabituation. Other research on fundamental relations between stimuli or behavioral patterns and central-nervous system activity tests the function of brain tissue (whether nourished or depleted) in performance, the mechanisms of sensory and perceptual information processing in the human visual system, and the neural mechanisms that link vision to motor activity. Memory formation is studied by the use of physiological stimuli, including both electroshock and drugs. Biological processes in memory are also the subject of an extended program of microbiological research.

The neurophysiology of attention is an area of special interest for several investigators. Their work extends from the study of the neurophysiological mechanisms underlying perception (including the regulation of sensory perception by cellular pools in the brain stem), to the ways in which brain processes underlying attention are affected by psychosis, aging, brain damage, and mental retardation. The functions of the inferior temporal cortex and the role of the hippocampus in problem-solving behavior are also being investigated. Studies of the psychophysiology of consciousness have

demonstrated that electrical activity of different parts of the brain, correlated with such autonomic activity as heart rate and muscle tension, is
responsive to conscious control. This finding may lead to many therapeutic
applications, particularly in treating psychosomatic illness. As mentioned
earlier, average evoked responses of schizophrenic, depressed, and hyperkinetic children are studied in relation to their behavior.

Other neurophysiological research with a specific behavioral tar-
get is directed to the underlying physiology and anatomy of aggression and
attack. In another study, a specialist in central nervous system control of
visceral processes has experimented, using animal models, with stereotactic
surgery for relief from pain, epilepsy, and other behavioral disorders.

*Sleeping and Dreaming.*   Some of the foregoing descriptions of
psychiatric research have referred to sleep phenomena. Although many scientists in mental health are interested in this new and exciting area, the number
of research psychiatrists and their associates responsible for the major developments in this field has been sufficiently limited to encourage a strongly
cohesive inter-relationship and necessarily broad research goals. Let us
identify the main problems under study.

The relatively recent discovery of REM (rapid eye movement)
sleep, during which most dreaming appears to occur, has served as a major
stimulus to monitoring sleep behavior. As a result, a territory of mental
and physical experience previously closed to behavioral research (with an
attraction and potential significance analogous to the anthropological discovery of an untouched Stone Age culture) has opened up. Sleep monitoring can now provide information on biochemical and neuronal processes,
giving access to the endocrinological and nervous systems and providing
specific comparative knowledge of the physiological mechanisms in various
levels of sleep and waking states. Laboratories equipped for this purpose
are now relatively common in psychiatric research programs.

Among the primary problems now under investigation are questions concerning natural functions. What are the normal patterns of REM
and non-REM sleep in healthy adults and children? How does the length
of the sleep period affect these patterns? Investigators are concerned with
minimal requirements in duration of REM and non-REM sleep, and with
the ways sleep deprivation affects waking performance. The tentative hypothesis of one investigator is that slow-wave (non-REM) sleep fulfills a
primarily biological need, whereas REM sleep fulfills a primarily psychological need.

The research broadens in one direction to the relation between
emotions during the waking hours and the duration and content of the
REM-period sleep. This relationship is tested by such experimental condi-

tions as the experience of stress films. Evidence from this kind of experimentation suggests that it may be possible to determine how defense mechanisms affect the production of dream content. Physiological measures of sleep-dream states gradually open up knowledge of the physiological and biochemical processes that underlie normal and disturbed patterns of sleep.

Additional knowledge of sleep physiology with its correlates, emotional or cognitive, is provided by psychopharmacological manipulation. The effects of alcohol and other drugs on sleep and subsequent performance are tested, as are the effects of dietary deprivation or imbalances.

Investigation of sleep patterns and affective disorders as well as the determination of biogenic amine metabolism relative to changes in sleep patterns extend the range of psychopharmacological knowledge and treatment. Much of this work, as one would expect, explores psychophysiological correlates in sleep by comparisons between normal and mentally ill subjects. Some implications of sleep research for the understanding of mental illness have been summarized by one investigator as follows:

> We feel that our work is extremely important in the area of mental health, particularly in the area of schizophrenic and depressive psychoses. We feel that certain aspects of the psychotic state must, by definition, include malfunctioning REM and [non]REM sleep mechanisms. . . .
> Many other areas should be touched by our work and should profit from it: the current treatment of sleep disorders; understanding the functional significance of sleep and, therefore, the care and treatment of insomnia; and, finally, a better understanding of the hygiene of sleep and the desired amount throughout life.

Knowledge of the relations between sleep patterns and neurophysiological and biochemical processes has been gained from a variety of experiments. It extends to the metabolism of biogenic amines in sleep, specifically to the effects of various naturally secreted hormones on dreaming and to the sleep correlates of amino acid deprivation.

In one study, the effect on dreaming of sensorimotor experience in waking hours is studied by observing patterns of movement in sleep. Movement is monitored by videotape in relation to EEG (electroencephalogram), EOG (electro-oculogram), and EMG (electromyelogram). Dream content is then correlated with specific movement patterns.

Electrical discharges recorded during sleep from the pontogeniculate-occipital area of cat brains have been compared with electrical activity from extra-ocular muscles in sleeping humans. The latter measurement may provide information concerning primary electrophysiological events during REM sleep. Studies based on this approach may be used to clarify the neurophysiological and biochemical processes that constitute the substrate of hallucinations and delusions.

One line of inquiry traces the function and the natural history of sleep in the development toward resourceful adaptation of the human organism, from the neonate through infancy. Disturbed sleep patterns in infancy, as demonstrated in brain-damaged and autistic children, are being compared with normal patterns.

*Personality Development and Social and Environmental Adaptation.*   The social factors underlying and shaping human behavior are under investigation by a diverse group of scientists whose subjects, methods, and chosen research problems are also highly varied. All, however, ultimately contribute to understanding the roots of psychopathological and normal adaptation.

An extensive program of research by one investigator traces how development of cognitive control relates to defense mechanisms and other aspects of personality organization. Data on 100 twins, 200 university students, and groups of impoverished black and white children are being analyzed for information on cognitive control in relation to vocational choice and on individual differences and educational processes.

Personality development in a socially and geographically isolated cultural environment is being studied through the field work of another investigator. To advance understanding of cultural components in personality development, he is devising objective scales to analyze projective test responses by American Indians.

A psychologist working with normal subjects and hospitalized patients is using multi-variant assessment techniques to study the phenomenon of attention. He is interested in the dimensions of habitual attention, the speed and character of attention shifts, and the relation of attentional behavior to internal stimuli and cognitive structure. This research may contribute to a clinically useful theory of attention, integrating physiological and clinical knowledge of this area with the viewpoint of ego psychology.

One research program on cognition is testing the hypothesis that we do not simply categorize incoming stimuli but actually establish an internal structure to handle incoming information. Cognitive mechanisms are thus studied in relation to auditory attention, visual memory, hallucinatory states, and levels of organization in reading and a variety of other perceptual and cognitive activities, both visual and auditory.

The province of another investigator is nonverbal communication: facial expression and body movement in relation to personality, culture, emotion, or stage of personality development. The studies of these subtle aspects of human communication have also been advanced by field work in a primitive culture, through special studies of children and by comparisons of behavior of mentally ill and normal adult subjects.

Other studies of basic behavioral processes include experimental work on how the organism copes with sensory deprivation (with emphasis on the configuration of physiological and mental responses) and a study of the subliminal effects produced by such varied states of consciousness as waking, dreaming, and hypnotic trance.

A sociologist is conducting a study designed to clarify the social causes of several states of stress and to demonstrate the role of various social relationships in ameliorating stress and aiding adaptive or coping behavior. Individuals for whom social circumstances have created unusual stress, such as divorced women and widows, are interviewed to see how they organize their lives to fulfill their personality needs.

A social psychologist whose present interest is how personality development is affected by special crises (domestic and occupational) that occur between the ages of 35 and 45, has also studied career development in the psychiatric setting, the authoritarian personality, and the organizational process. Similar work has been done by a sociologist who has been particularly interested in comparing doctoral candidates in biochemistry and residents in internal medicine and psychiatry.


## Child Development


Research in child development, which began as a particular concern of psychologists, now has a strong psychiatric cast. The child development research endeavor supported by the Research Development Program is carried out by a diverse group of investigators that includes psychiatrists, psychologists, biochemists, sociologists, a physiologist, and a pediatrician with some psychiatric training.

The scientists conducting developmental studies may be divided into two groups: those who are concerned primarily with normal developmental processes (whether physiological, emotional, cognitive, or social), and those who focus on psychopathological behavior. (There is some overlap in their concerns; for example, one investigator who began with an extensive inquiry into normal adolescence has turned to the case history and culture study of adolescent delinquents.)

The overall objective of the first group is to discover the complex of factors that contribute to healthy child development. In other words, they wish to find out how resourceful adaptation occurs. Areas of investigation span the life experiences from the prenatal period through adolescence (with emphasis on the early years) and include the sensorimotor, perceptual, and affective experiences of the neonate; the crucial mother-child interaction of infancy; and the physical, cognitive, and social experiences of later childhood. Scientists studying normal development often collect data from sustained structured observation in natural (or simulated natural) settings rather than using operant conditioning or observation of responses to controlled stimuli. The neonatal and early infancy periods, which receive considerable research attention, are studied particularly with an eye toward sensorimotor and cognitive functions, perceptual behavior, and the neurophysiological correlates of behavior.

The following rationale by one researcher of his studies in the area of early development typifies the current viewpoint of many of his colleagues:

> Research on human infants has, in the past decade, appreciably changed our view of the capacities and developmental potentialities of the young baby. We no longer see him as an amorphous, vegetative being, as earlier viewpoints characteristically did.
>
> Now that we know that he is capable of sophisticated perceptual discrimination, that he can learn conditioning tasks, that even his biological sleep-wake rhythms are to some extent under control of caretaker conditions, we must raise new questions about the nature of earliest experience on later development. To me the connection of these issues to the mental health of children, to problems of education and cognitive development, and to the nature of family life—particularly in those segments of the population where family life is most threatened—are self-evident. Ultimately, we must be able to plan programs that are preventive and educational rather than restitutive and therapeutic. . . .

The more extended studies of childhood and puberty by program participants include topics such as sleep development in normal children (compared with brain-damaged or institutionalized children); the growth of speech and speech mechanisms in normal and abnormal development; the comparative neurological development of normals and the neurologically handicapped; development of affective and cognitive behavior; and psychobiological development considered cross-culturally.

Of the scientists who focus on psychopathological behavior in childhood, more than half study, in clinical settings, the psychological, physical, and social components of disturbed behavior (from severe psychosis to learning disabilities). The remainder work in laboratories with animal subjects and are concerned mainly with abnormal development of the brain, the central nervous system, and the endocrinological systems in relation to psychiatric disturbances.

In research on the psychopathology of childhood, other investigators study children with specific symptoms or syndromes and experiment to discover effective methods of treatment. For example, several studies of autistic children have focused variously on family background, sleep disturbance, language behavior, and the possibility of a chronic brain syndrome. Psychotherapy, behavior therapy, and the use of teaching machines are the treatment procedures under investigation.

Among the special targets of study are children who are schizophrenic, depressed, or hyperkinetic. An investigator working with children with the latter problem has gleaned appreciable social and behavioral data; his search now continues on the biochemical front:

> I have maintained a program of research into the natural history of the hyperactive child, an important problem for elementary school education since it is estimated that one out of ten grade-school boys has handicaps in learning because of it. I have accomplished the following: a description of the hyperactive child syndrome, directing attention to the fact that hyperactive children often present antisocial behavior such as lying and stealing and showing that accidentally poisoned boys frequently turn out to be hyperactive grade-schoolers; a follow-up study of hyperactive children, which shows that as teen-agers they continue to have the basic problems of restlessness, distractability, impulsiveness, irritability, a very low interest in school, and a poor opinion of themselves. In this last study we found that a number of the hyperactive children could be classified as delinquents when they were teen-agers, and that a minority were sociopaths.
>
> My most recent study of hyperactive children seems to be the most significant. I have studied the families of a group of hyperactive children and compared them with the families of a suitable group of control children. We have found that the fathers and grandfathers of hyperactive children are significantly more likely to be alcoholics or to be problem drinkers than the corresponding relatives of control children. Furthermore the evidence suggests that the alcoholic fathers of hyperactive children were probably hyperactive children themselves. There is also significant association between hyperactive children and parents who are either alcoholic, sociopathic, or hysteric.
>
> I feel that this last study is a very important lead for further research. Clearly it is necessary to confirm the findings with a larger study; assuming that the findings were confirmed, we would have a clue to antecedents of alcoholism and a group in which we could investigate the inheritance or social transmission of a specific temperament.
>
> My major interest now is in finding a biochemical correlate to variations in the temperament of children; the particular temperament that I am interested in, namely the hyperactive child, seems to be related to the massive problems of learning difficulties in

grade school, delinquency, and alcoholism. I hope, therefore, that
my future research will contribute to understanding the biological
aspects of these problems.

Other foci of research attention are children who suffer from congenital
defects (including brain damage and genetic deficiencies); and emotionally
disturbed adolescents. Investigative techniques include neurophysiological
and chemical measurements, family studies, and experimental treatment
(which includes family counseling and psychotherapy, group treatment in
a residential center, and behavior therapy). Drug treatment is used with
some children suffering from mongolism and hyperkinetic behavior.

For investigators working in experimental school situations with
children suffering from learning disabilities, experimental techniques are
both educational and psychopharmacological. One worker reports the following progress in school-related problems:

> My program of research attempts to determine the effects of drugs
> on learning and behavior in children with school failure and dis-
> turbances of behavior, and to investigate physiological causes and
> correlates of these problems.
>
> At present, the research is focusing on the use of cortical-evoked
> responses and other physiologic measures (such as autonomic
> function) in defining certain groups of children who have a bio-
> logical basis for their learning and behavioral disabilities. Published
> studies indicate promising leads in identifying some children who
> fail to read or learn in school—who have abnormalities in brain
> function not detected by other methods. For instance, the data
> indicate that some poor readers who come from families of poor
> readers have abnormalities of visual-evoked response in the left
> parietal areas of the brain. Concurrent pharmacological treatment
> studies have also shown that these bioelectric phenomena can be
> significantly altered by psychoactive drugs.
>
> A major portion of the research is the investigation of drugs that
> have therapeutic application in the control of disruptive behavior.
> A recently completed study comparing two widely used sympathomi-
> metic amines (methylphenidate and dextroamphetamine) showed
> a clear therapeutic benefit from both drugs, but one of the drugs
> (methylphenidate) produced more change in certain cognitive tests
> and fewer side effects. These findings have considerable practical
> importance in the pediatric use of these agents. Other drug studies
> have dealt with control of behavior in children with violent behavior
> and antisocial behavior; some promising leads for further research
> have resulted from these studies (for example, diphenylhydantoin
> appears to be useful in a small sub-group of children with violent
> temper tantrums). New drugs (such as magnesium pemoline hy-
> droxide) are also being tested for possible effects on behavior
> control and learning. These are all carefully placebo-controlled,
> double-blind studies. . . .

The work encompassed in these studies has immediate practical relevance in several areas: it serves to establish the degree of usefulness and limits of psychoactive agents in the clinical management of children with a variety of behavior and learning defects. It may lead to methods for early detection and classification of one of the world's most significant public health problems, reading failure. The work has implications for the causes of violent and antisocial behavior and gives useful information on some proposed somatic treatments for these conditions. From a theoretical and scientific point of view, the investigation of brain function and its relation to cognitive function in children may provide basic information on the role of genetic, neurophysiologic, and biochemical substrates of children's behavior, especially communication skills such as reading.

Cultural studies of child development are being conducted in deprived socioeconomic settings. Particular attention is given to contrasts between the play behavior of ghetto and nonghetto children, the cognitive capacity of environmentally deprived children as manifested in language capacity, and the effectiveness of individualized language teaching. One striking finding has been that regardless of racial background, the same factors in the childhood environment can be used to predict later success and occupations as well as such social and psychological disorders as drug addiction, alcoholism, and criminal behavior.

Investigators conducting laboratory studies explore the development of the central nervous system at organismic and cellular levels and trace the developmental impact on neonatal animals of interventions such as deprivation, shock, or stress of various kinds, testing effects on both physiological structures and adaptive behavioral capabilities. One investigator described his studies in this area as follows:

> My research is directed at the problem of how early experiences alter the process of mammalian development after birth so as to produce adults with maladaptive emotional and physiological responses. My strategy is to focus on a relatively easily studied model system in a rapidly developing mammal and to use the experimental method to discover fundamental biological mechanisms and the principles by which they alter the outcome of development in this system.
>
> The neural regulation of cardiac function in the laboratory rat was chosen for several reasons. The functioning of this system can be readily quantified and recorded from unrestrained animals of all ages, and this system is influenced by the highest levels of the central nervous system. Furthermore, some adult rats are susceptible to cardiac arrhythmias and sudden cardiac arrest under stress, as are some humans.
>
> The first step was to investigate the stages by which the organism

develops cardiac responses to environmental stimulation. This work uncovered a stage in the second week of postnatal life when cardiac regulation is organized in a radically different way from the adult. Next, I was able to show that separation of the infant rat from its mother during this critical early period produced a massive physiological response in the pups. Resting heart rates fell 40 to 50 percent in a 12-hour period. Present work suggests the exciting possibility that neural development in this system may be immediately responsive to altered levels of nutrition in the normal range. I am currently trying to ascertain the mechanism by which developing neural systems respond to short-term changes in nutritional intake. . . .

This research bears directly on the problems generated in our country today by the impact of the social and inanimate environment on the development of children and the long-term effects on brain and behavior that will be evident in adults. Specifically, we have good reason to suspect that cardiovascular disease is related to our way of life, and yet the role of early experiences in determining susceptibility to these illnesses is wholly unknown today. This kind of research into the effects of early experience on disease susceptibility promises to open up a whole new area of preventive medicine and offers the hope of controlling many illnesses for which no effective therapy can be found.

In another line of study, children's capacity for resistance to disease is correlated with normal ego development and the capacity for social experience.

Several of the investigators dealing with early development are concerned with gonadal function and development, with neuroendocrinological processes in sex behavior, and with the effects of normal and abnormal production of hormones such as androgen on the development of sex-specific behavior. In a more behaviorally oriented investigation of sexual deviation, one investigator has conducted family studies designed to facilitate early detection and treatment:

My research is directed to understanding the etiology of various forms of atypical sexual behavior during adulthood.

I am studying a group of preadolescent boys whose behavior is very similar to the retrospectively described boyhood behavior of adult homosexuals, trans-sexuals, and transvestites. These boys' behavior includes frequent dressing in girls' clothes, a strong preference for playing with girls, a strong preference for girls' games, and overt statements of wanting to be a girl. The boys are being extensively studied through interviews, psychological tests, standardized play situations, and films. Their parents are being studied by individual and joint interviews, under a variety of experimental settings, as couples and with their sons. Preliminary data on a continuing longitudinal study of similar boys plus other follow-up studies indicate that most of these boys, untreated, will grow up to be trans-sexual, homosexual, or transvestic. On the basis of findings from the above research evaluations, programs of treatment are being instituted with the younger boys currently under study who are experiencing social distress due to their atypical behavior.

Future plans include systematic comparisons of several intra-familial factors in families in which a boy is manifesting atypical behavior and in families in which typical sexuality is emerging. Arrangements are being made for longitudinal periodic evaluation of the boys currently under study, with follow-up through adolescence and into adulthood.

To date there has been generated the largest single sample of boys with an atypical sexual identity and their families. A more detailed behavioral description of these boys, their parents, and patterns of family interaction is being gathered than has previously been available.

Population surveys indicate there are 6 million adult Americans who are homosexuals. Some of these persons are in considerable emotional conflict because of their sexual behavior. Psychiatric efforts directed at sexual reorientation during adulthood for those who want reorientation have fallen considerably short of expectations. Evidence indicates that the earlier diagnosis of such behavior is made and the earlier psychiatric intervention instituted, the greater the likelihood of preventing future distress. Additionally, as more is learned about the etiology of atypical sexuality from direct family study during the persons' childhood, the more will also be learned about typical patterns of sexual expression.

Chapter 2 has presented a glimpse of the diversity and range of studies conducted by participants in the Research Development Program. The quotations were chosen to represent a sampling of this diversity, which ranges from basic laboratory studies to clinical research, from biochemistry to sociology and anthropology, and from studies of normal phenomena and processes to investigations of pathology in animals and humans.

Given the very short history of scientific psychiatric research and the complexity of human behavior to which it is ultimately addressed, it would be premature to expect many dramatic clinically applicable findings to have emerged yet from the grantees' studies. In most areas of scientific research, unless there is extraordinary luck, a certain critical mass of basic information must be accumulated (usually quite slowly and painstakingly) before there is likely to be a breakthrough. The Research Development Program has supported individual men rather than research projects, partly because many of these studies require a lifetime of slow, careful study and may not show results in the normal course of short grant periods.

Most of the grantees, whether psychiatrists or other scientists, are doing the basic intellectual spadework that is essential for progress in mental health research. They are studying basic functions of the nervous system; devising methods for analyzing and evaluating various forms of therapy; observing the natural history of psychopathology; or finding and working with animal subjects that can serve as substitutes for humans in experimental studies. Although none of these studies, by itself, may necessarily result directly in better treatment of schizophrenia or depression, for example, together they provide the intellectual foundations for improved practice and may contribute in the long run to significant clinical applications. The following examples illustrate only a few of the promising directions of recent work.

A number of studies have yielded or promise to yield provocative clues to the causes and treatment of mental illness. Some findings of direct clinical relevance have already emerged. In many instances, these findings have been based on recognition that many psychiatric problems can be overcome by techniques, both investigative and therapeutic, derived from other disciplines. For example, one psychiatrist is developing new treatments for stuttering as well as for chronic, severe sexual inhibition in married women (two disorders that have had, according to that researcher, a poor prognosis with other methods of treatment). His therapeutic methods are based on learning principles and rely in part on desensitization techniques whereby patients learn to relax in the presence of feared stimuli. Stutterers are helped also by wearing a tiny hearing-aid-like metronome that helps them pace their speech.

In a related study exploring the uses of desensitization therapy, another grantee has been able to reduce patients' phobic behavior by using a computer that functions as a therapist. This grantee reports that automated techniques are as successful as a human therapist in reducing fear. He is also exploring specific patterns of changed physiological responses associated with successful treatment.

As mentioned in the preceding section on research in psychosomatic medicine, several investigators are exploring the extent to which functions of the autonomic nervous system (such as regulation of blood pressure, heart rate, and gastric secretions) can come under conscious control. (The therapeutic applications of these techniques to hypertension, heart disease, and ulcers, among others, are obvious.) In addition, one investigator is studying how the brain's electrical activity can be modified by conscious control. Aspects of the brain's electrical activity, detected by electrodes, can be fed back to subjects as a tone of variable loudness that they can modify by changing their state of mind. The investigator is studying the application of this promising technique to a number of mental health problems such as chronic anxiety, stomach ulcers, migraine, and chronic tension headaches.

Research concerned with the biochemical bases of mental illness has yielded a number of promising avenues for therapy. For example, through advanced biochemical techniques, a student of endocrine disturbance in depression has been able to demonstrate significant disturbances of adrenocortical function in a substantial number of depressed patients. The precise clinical features of depressive illness associated with this endocrine disturbance have also been identified. Growth hormone secretion also appears to be abnormal in a number of depressed patients, particularly in the diurnal patterns of secretion. This investigator and another awardee at the same institution are studying the possibility that the sleep disturbance seen in depression may be linked to this abnormal secretion pattern. The effects of lithium carbonate therapy on endocrine function are also under investigation. Out of these studies is emerging a clearer picture of central nervous system abnormalities (particularly disturbance of the hypothalamus, which directly regulates hormonal activity) that may underlie many affective disorders as well as psychosomatic illness. With such knowledge, it may then be possible to devise therapeutic measures that can reverse these pathological processes.

Following the same general logic are studies directed to elucidating the disturbances of brain chemistry that underlie psychotic behavior, particularly schizophrenia. Studies have been focused particularly on the action of naturally occurring chemicals, the biogenic amines (including catecholamines, serotonin, and histamine), which are concentrated in brain areas having to do with emotional functions. They are also examining the way these natural chemicals interact with drugs, especially psychedelics like LSD, to produce and alter behavior. Several benefits can accrue from such studies, including (1) understanding how brain chemistry relates to behavior, both normal and abnormal, and (2) understanding how psychotropic drugs exert their clinical actions so that new therapeutic agents can be predicted and developed to alleviate naturally occurring psychoses and the disturbed behavior produced by drug abuse.

Research Development Program grantees have developed the following productive leads. One investigator has devised a molecular model that can predict the action of a number of psychoactive drugs. Potential benefits of l-amphetamine for Parkinson's disease and for hyperkinetic behavior in children have thus been predicted and found. This same investigator has more recently discovered the specific sites in the brain (particularly in the corpus striatum, which is involved in integrating perceptual information and motor activity) where opiate drugs produce their effects; he has shown that the clinical potency of such drugs in man can be predicted from their binding activity in brain tissue. In addition to shedding light on the physical basis of opiate addiction (and perhaps other forms of addiction), this study provides an effective method for rapidly testing the strength of new opiate drugs and antagonists.

Several valuable avenues of research that may aid in the early detection and prevention of psychopathology (as well as understanding the preconditions for psychological strength and resiliency) are concerned with the early development of children. A rather serendipitous and extremely practical finding has emerged from one grantee's study of the effects of substandard environmental conditions on the development of the immature central nervous system. In the course of studying how blood concentrations of certain amino acids affect normal brain development and function, he discovered that relatively mild and transient elevations of glutamic acid can rapidly destroy certain parts of the hypothalamus and possibly other parts of the brain. Since glutamic acid (monosodium glutamate, or MSG) is a common additive in foods, including baby food, its effects on fetal and young children clearly deserve study, a message communicated by this researcher to numerous responsible federal agencies and commissions. The destructive effects of glutamic acid on the developing brain, at least in infant animals, are greatest in those deficient in vitamin $B_6$—as are many of the world's poor and undernourished. Thus, these findings may have particular relevance to the diets of people whose children are already developmentally at risk from other aspects of the culture of poverty. This study has contributed to greater awareness of the need for testing food additives as they affect the developing nervous system; it has also generated new recommendations for food safety.

Another grantee, who is well known for his studies of the early roots of intelligence and motivation, has developed six scales of psychological development in infancy that promise a new approach to assessing development and intelligence at very young ages (presumably when intervention may improve developmental patterns). He is also conducting a long-term study of the psychological development of infants in orphanages when various types of psychological enrichment are provided to preserve and enhance the infants' intellectual development.

A student of the early years (who for 20 years had studied schizophrenia in adults) is concentrating on identifying children presumably vulnerable to schizophrenia (due to genetic predisposition, familial social pathology, or poor sociocultural environment). He has been comparing their behavior with presumably normal children, developing measures to identify patterns of competence and incompetence, and testing new modes of intervention to help "immunize" high-risk or vulnerable children against later disorder. He is also studying the adaptive potential of inner-city "invulnerable" children who, despite the disadvantages of their environments, possess "strengths of ego and will." Among the provocative leads to emerge from this study is the possibility that aspects of peer play may provide subtle indices of early failures of adaptation that otherwise might go unheeded, at least by adults.

Most of the studies just cited seem likely to lead to relatively clear-cut preventive or therapeutic applications now or in the near future. Yet the ultimate impact of these and other investigations (such as many of those cited earlier in the chapter) is almost impossible to predict. To some extent, then, as those responsible for the Research Development Program have recognized, their long-term support of promising scientists is a gamble. As one chairman of a prominent department of psychiatry put it:

> If one seriously believes, as we do, that advance in health care cannot take place without new discoveries, one is convinced that the investment in a manpower base from which such discoveries may come is a solid [one]. No one career recipient can produce guaranteed results. Discovery is always a matter, to a certain extent, of good fortune and rare combinations of talent.

Judging by the research contributions of Research Development Program grantees, good fortune and talent have combined often. Psychiatry and, ultimately, the patients the profession serves must benefit, now and in the future.

Chapters 3 and 4 will explore, largely from the perspective of the scientist-grantees themselves, some of the conditions that help or hinder the growth of their scientific abilities and productivity.

# Research in the Psychiatric Setting

## 3

*The Psychiatrist as Researcher*

Research of the types described in the preceding chapter is relatively new in psychiatry. As a full-time activity it still engages a minuscule (but growing) segment of the profession. To psychiatrists trained and working in traditional medical schools and departments of psychiatry, research can still appear to be an irrelevant and even risky way to spend one's time. In fact, there is a long and honorable tradition in psychiatry that reinforces these attitudes. (See Chapter 6, History of the Research Development Program.) The Research Development Program (particularly in its initial form as the Career Investigator Grant program) was specifically designed to overcome some of the deterrents to research and to encourage able young psychiatrists to receive the training and experience needed for research competence and a commitment to a research career. This chapter will explore some of the strains inherent in psychiatry that tend to inhibit research; it will document the experiences of a number of psychiatrist grantees who have coped with such strains, usually quite successfully, with the help of the program. As the following pages will show, progress in psychiatric research can be stimulated by outside influences such as the Research Development Program, but it still depends largely on the willingness of a few devoted men and women to make personal and economic sacrifices (compared with their colleagues in private practice) to pursue scientific truth.

*Psychiatry and Research.* Psychiatry appears to have been slow to develop a research base compared with other branches of medicine.

Possibly problems of dealing with mental disorder are more complicated, more difficult, and possibly even of a different type than the problems in other branches of medicine. They simply may not, by their nature, yield to the same pattern of differential diagnosis, isolation of etiology, and determination of the procedures of cure. The medically trained psychiatric resident often faces this head-on, as this psychiatric researcher did:

> During my internship in medicine. . . I saw a large number of patients with a wide variety of medical illnesses. Some had failing hearts, some bad livers, others had lung diseases, and so forth. But in working up individual patients thoroughly I came across healthy "parts" in almost all of them. By listening to hundreds of healthy hearts in my patients ill with other diseases, for example, I came to know what a healthy heart sounded like through the stethoscope, looked like on the EKG, and so on. When I stumbled on a bad heart, I recognized it in comparison to what I knew was a good heart. The sound was different, it was shaped differently on the X ray, its electrical pattern looked different on the EKG, and so forth. It was this model of continuously focusing on the healthy organ as a baseline for recognition of an unhealthy one that made sense to me in the clinical practice of medicine.
>
> Then I came to psychiatry. My first year of residency was a nightmare. Wherever I looked, all I saw was abnormalcy (so I was told by my supervisors.) Psychopathology was not as considerate as liver disease. It did not leave healthy areas side by side with pathological ones. It intrudes somewhat in all areas of the personality. Thus each patient was in *all* ways unique. Issues of "what is normalcy?" "does it really exist?" thoroughly confused me and left me floating, dependent on my supervisor to inform me how far off from normalcy this or that patient was. I could find little clinical baseline data on normalcy. My desire was to leave psychiatry, which I did briefly. Dr. ———, however, convinced me to return, noting that it would all clear up in due course.
>
> As a matter of fact, he was right. I was fascinated by the problems presented by each individual patient—by the experiences of dynamic evaluation—and forgot about issues of normalcy. If it didn't bother others, why should it bother me? Clinical [psychiatry] was the science of guided intuition, and to hell with the rest. It was fun, and people did get better.

The problem, however, is that people do get better, sometimes, under psychoanalytic treatment, with electro-convulsive treatment, with the ministrations of the Indian medicine man or the practitioner of voodoo, and the simple passage of time. Given the difficulty of diagnosis and recognition and the nonspecificity of treatment procedures, it is understandable that some bright young psychiatrists might conclude that mental illness itself is a myth to be treated with myths rather than medicine. However, a violent schizophrenic is no myth, nor is a severely depressed person, nor an autistic child. Each presents a serious human problem. Each demands hope of alleviation of that problem. Each must be approached by the dedicated psychiatrist with the techniques at hand.

The difficulties inherent in the field of mental illness and psychiatry are of such magnitude that Shepherd (1971) says: "The precise role of psychiatry as a branch of medicine has still to be established and accepted (p. 218)." The lack of a set of medical procedures that are clearly and demonstrably superior to myth and magic, combined with emphasis on developing self-confidence in medical training as a prerequisite for assuming life-and-death responsibility for patients, has placed the psychiatrist in an exceedingly difficult position. Of all the medical specialists, he must deal with the most common human problems with the least demonstrably effective tools. It is not surprising that for many psychiatrists, the need to feel and act competent overshadows the need to know.

There are other factors inherent in psychiatry that also serve to retard research progress. Many of these appear to be chronically in conflict with the research endeavor. For example, departments of psychiatry do not intrinsically provide fertile ground for the growth and cultivation of science. The psychiatrist, whose primary motivation is to alleviate the distress of mental disorder, is impatient with the impracticality and apparent irrelevance of basic research. His responsibility for and occupation with patient management consume his time and energy to the exclusion of the remote and abstract. His need for self-confidence in the practice of his skills leaves little room for doubt and questioning. Given the primarily clinical orientation of departments of psychiatry and their leading members, some observers feel that maintaining a good clinical service and training facility is nearly incompatible with simultaneously maintaining a good research and research training facility.

Another source of difficulty arises from what Albee (1970), discussing clinical psychology, has portrayed as the difference between the scientist and the professional practitioner. He says:

> *Science* is open and its knowledge is public. . . . A free-wheeling spirit of incisive mutual and self-criticism, replication, debate, and argument over procedures, findings, and interpretation of data is ever-present (p. 1075).

On the other hand:

> A *profession* must jealously guard its secrets! Historically, one of the hallmarks of a profession has been the privacy of its knowledge. If the knowledge of the professional, his techniques, and his

skills are available to anyone and could be performed by anyone, a profession would disintegrate. Secrecy and mystery are essential (p. 1075).

Albee's analysis leads him to conclude that there is a fundamental incompatibility of the roles of scientist and professional in one individual.

Albee's conclusion, in an absolute form, is obviously incorrect. There are now a number of successful scientist-practitioners in psychiatry, in many branches of clinical medicine as well as in clinical psychology. But it is unquestionably a dual role that is difficult to maintain, as the comments of Research Development Program grantees on the following pages will show; for many individuals, it may be impossible, whether or not for the reasons Albee proposes.

To explore some of the personal effects of participation in psychiatric research, in March 1972 Dr. Boothe sent an informal letter to a small sample (14) of research psychiatrists who had received Research Development Program awards for periods of from 6 to 16 years. They were asked to describe what the award has meant in the context of personal interests and professional circumstances.

The replies to this request were personal, rich, and varied. Yet certain common themes emerged repeatedly. Judging by comments made by other grantees, the remarks of the 13 who replied reflect the general experiences of most psychiatrists in the program and perhaps of research psychiatrists in general.

*Facilitating Research.* The dominant theme of the replies concerned the crucial role of the Research Development Program (through its full-time, long-term salary support) in enabling grantees to make a total commitment to research. As one investigator noted:

> For me, as a psychiatrist with clinical and psychoanalytic training, a continuing and primary commitment to research would have been just unthinkable and out of the question completely without the award. True, I had been engaged as a research psychiatrist from 1954 to 1962, supported through specific project funding. However, the instability and discontinuity inherent in that avenue as a source of personal income was too painfully apparent to me, by the end of that period, to consider continuing on the basis of project support. The almost nonexistent institutional support for medical school faculty at that time required one's major investment in clinical practice.

Many other respondents mentioned the dual detriments to full-time research: first, unstable and discontinuous research project support that had to be continually sought from sources outside the institution and, second, the implicit demands of the medical system that faculty members justify their presence (and earn tenure) through clinical service, teaching, and administrative activities.

Two of the respondents speculated on the alternate routes their careers might have taken had the awards not been available when they were. Said one:

> The Research Career Award has, I think, been crucial in my professional and personal life. Of course as a scientist I do not have control data—that is, where I would be now or how I would have gotten there without this career program. However, there is nobody in our department who has been able to devote himself primarily to academic psychiatry who has not been supported by this program. It is possible that I could have received salary support from research grants and could have developed a similar professional career; however, the personal financial insecurity that this course would have entailed would perhaps have made me assume other kinds of responsibilities in the medical school and hospital and have pulled me away from a strictly academic career.

The other respondent observed that:

> I would like to start with the emphatic statement that the Research Development Program in a very concrete and real sense determined my career in medicine. . . . Throughout college and medical school my eventual plan was to do research. At the time of graduation from medical school, however, I was faced with the decision of taking a Ph.D. in neurophysiology (laboratory science) or further training in psychiatry. After doing a year in neurophysiology, I decided to go into psychiatry because I wanted to work directly with human beings. At the time I saw no clear path to doing research that would also utilize my medical training and at the same time permit me to pursue psychiatric training. With the encouragement of Dr. ———, who called my attention to the Research Development Program, I was able to undertake training in psychiatric research under the program, which crystallized my career. It is conceivable that I would have found a way of combining clinical psychiatry and research; but the fate of many of my colleagues who expressed an interest in research and have ended up in full-time psychiatric practice has left me wondering whether I would have been able to withstand the many pressures to continue in clinical work without the support of a Career Grant.

The young would-be researcher is frequently faced with strong pressure to engage in clinical activities. As his research career advances, however, other pressures are added that seem calculated to deter him from a full-time commitment to research—most notably, academic or clinical administrative duties. For example, in most psychiatric settings, clinical services are delivered by nurses, aides, social workers, clinical psychologists, residents, and medical students. The trained psychiatrist, by contrast, is usually in an administrative position with responsibility for those psychiatric service personnel and the clinics and wards in which they work. As observed by several grantees, the award has not only supported them to do full-time research but has provided an alternative self-definition that allows them to resist distractions such as administrative responsibility:

> The matter is rather simple. At present, I feel quite strongly motivated to continue, perhaps for the duration of my professional career, in a position with a total commitment to research. Practically speaking, this means that I am not particularly eager to assume more administrative positions, such as a departmental chairmanship. Without the Career Award, I don't think I would have such a firm motivation. Academic life, especially in private universities, is always tenuous in its financial aspects. People in clinical departments who are doing research feel under a constant pressure to secure grants not only for their research but to pay their own salaries. This is a hell of a way for people with such advanced training and talents to subsist. I am sure that it is for this reason that many of the best researchers in clinical departments move at an early stage into departmental chairmanships. Too often they do this despite the fact that they would *a priori* have greatly preferred to remain in research. Because people's inclinations and skills generally go hand in hand, what frequently results is that a highly productive scientist is saddled with an administrative post he does not really want and is perhaps not ideally suited to handle —[the] Peter Principle. I think the Research Development Program is a powerful force militating against such silliness. . . . If administrative, teaching, and clinical activities are thrust at me to such an extent that they might interfere with my research, I simply reply that I am being paid to do science.

Another investigator, also alluding to the Peter Principle in academic medicine, went on to emphasize how recognition for the researcher role helps him to resist administrative and other distractions:

> In my own situation and from the observation of others in situations similar to my own, I have come to the not very novel conclusion that once a person attains a degree of "visibility" through his research efforts, there are powerful forces set into motion that tend to prevent him from doing further research. Administrative duties within the school (committees, interviewing) and commitments to the outside (seminar presentations, writing chapters and reviews, study sections, membership on editorial

boards) serve to separate the researcher from direct on-line participation in research. Each distraction in itself may represent a worthwhile and important endeavor. However, taken together these
various functions can effectively use up the time formerly given to
creative thought and research.

In my own case, aside from personal motivation, I feel that
support through the NIMH Research Development Program has
served as the principal barrier against total distraction from research.
This works in both obvious and subtle ways. Not only does the
financial support from the program provide a considerable degree
of independence from local pressure but, more important, one is
thought of in the "role" of a researcher. Of course, one cannot
exclude activities outside of research and in fact this would lead
to an undesirable kind of isolation. The difference the program
makes is where the line is drawn in choosing among the many
potential and worthwhile outside activities.

Despite whatever financial and moral support the program may
provide for individual researchers, they nonetheless must struggle actively
to keep their time free for research. The preceding respondent, for example,
observed that it had been a constant struggle for him to keep such outside
functions within manageable limits. Part of the problem stems from the
fact that the research scientist is constantly swimming against the tide of
social and professional expectations and is made to feel guilty if he appears
to abandon his professional responsibilities:

> Because research has always given me an enormous amount of
> satisfaction, I have resisted the accumulation of major administrative
> responsibilities such as being chairman of a department, although
> the evasion does cause me an occasional pang of conscience.

Related to the freedom from administrative and other academic
duties is the independence Research Development Program grantees feel
from the local political pressures of their sponsoring departments:

> The program has allowed me to be independent of the various power
> factions within both the department and the school, and thus I have
> been able to exert my influence in favor of scientific objectivity and
> skepticism notwithstanding various sorts of disapproval from supe-
> riors. This financial underpinning of my academic freedom allowed
> me also to be independent not only of the department but in the
> various controversies raging in the school as a whole. Whether my
> independence served for better or for worse is for others to judge,
> but I think that I could not have felt as independent if it had not
> been for the career program. . . . In summary, the career program
> has facilitated my making whatever scientific contributions I have
> been able to produce in the area of mental health; in addition, it

has allowed me to become . . . an ombudsman for objective scholarship in the behavioral sciences.

For many Research Development Program grantees, their special freedom from conventional academic responsibilities brings with it a
concomitant sense of responsibility:

> Freedom to work on problems of interest and exemption from ad-
> ministrative duties is not an unmixed blessing. It is accompanied by
> a deeply felt sense of obligation to make maximum use of the op-
> portunity afforded and to contribute as much as possible. I can only
> hope that my work so far has justified the confidence placed in me.

This discussion of the impact of the award has so far emphasized
freedom from various factors, whether incessant grant applications and
anxiety, clinical demands, or administrative politics and responsibility. But
equally significant has been the positive aspect: by providing investigators
with a relatively long and stable period of support with the promise of an
even longer subsequent period of support, the program has encouraged
many grantees to pursue problems that might otherwise have appeared too
risky or unconventional for them to explore. In other words, many investigators have followed their own interests and leads rather than studying
problems likely to yield quick results in time to meet short-term grant
reviews:

> The possibility of pursuing and gradually extending my own
> hunches about investigating the organization of different infant
> caretaker systems—especially the role of temporal factors in the
> development of the infant's various specific functions under these
> different conditions—would have been simply out of the question
> without personal support. The reason for this is that I would never
> have felt confident enough to propose specific projects stemming
> from this viewpoint without a slow period of preliminary work in
> which ideas and empirical feedback could proceed together. Pre-
> maturely crystalizing ideas into a formal research application, which
> then may be rejected, can eliminate such ideas from active develop-
> ment. Furthermore, the reduced administrative teaching and clinical
> responsibilities that the award has made possible have permitted me
> to continue thinking along certain lines, reading, and trying to in-
> tegrate experience and data in new work from the various levels:
> clinical, conceptual, and empirical-observational. For [the] . . . per-
> son who is without support necessary for relative autonomy, the
> work of crossing boundaries of competence takes either great self-
> confidence or great daring. . . .

Another grantee, looking back at his plunge into risky research, found that over the years his seemingly eccentric research has become a more popular area of concern:

> I recently reviewed some memoranda written more than 10 years ago in which I outlined some of the problems on which I wanted to work; problems that did not fall within any one established discipline. I remember that at the time friends and colleagues urged me to reject these problems lying on the interface of disciplines in favor of more traditional concerns that, in their view, would further my professional career.
>
> As a result of 10 years of support from the Research Development Program, I was fortunate [enough to be able] to devote myself to working on these problems. I find, at this time, that many of these concerns are more in the mainstream.

As one psychiatrist-researcher observed, the fact of doing research full time and receiving continuous support to do it affects the character and quality of the research itself:

> The Research Development [Program] award has allowed me to develop and use my particular talents and interests to make the maximum personal contribution to psychiatry and to my sponsoring department. This would not have been possible without the award simply because time would not have been available. I believe that serious research must be done on a full-time basis. If it is done part time, the researcher is almost certain to limit himself to the skills and techniques that he brought with him to the job. He may do worthwhile work, but it will be within a limited context, and it is more likely to amount to refinement than innovation.

According to many of the respondents, the presence of the Research Development Program has had a significant impact not only on themselves, but on their sponsoring departments as well. (For further discussion of departmental impact, see the beginning of Chapter 5.) Over the years, several grantees have observed laboratories devoted to psychiatric research or have led in establishing them. The program has often supported more than one individual in a department, leading to a special sort of spirit and sense of identity; it has fostered recognition of awardees as honored individuals who can enhance both the stature and the state of knowledge of the sponsoring department. For example, as one awardee noted:

> [My] sense of identity [as a researcher] was further reinforced by having [Drs. ———— and ————], both career awardees, join the same department at the same time, creating a sense of esprit [de corps] and commitment to research, as well as a feeling of pride in a new department with so many career researchers on board.

This investigator, like several others, alluded to the sense of pride the award gave him and the moral support it provided during moments of discouragement:

> I felt very lonely and unappreciated at times at [my previous research institution], and the sense of status I felt from receiving the award was very important to me. . . . [A corollary grant to the career award] meant a lot to me, but so did the feeling that the Research Development Program was a source of moral support in tough times. . . . Indeed, every so often when I get discouraged, I look through the list of Career Investigators, and I decide I must be good if I am in such distinguished company!

Another psychiatrist-researcher, alluding to his own sense of pride in having received the award observed that:

> I have always considered it to be a distinction and an honor to be a recipient of the award. This was particularly true earlier in my career and I still list it under "Honors and Awards" on my curriculum vitae.

As awardees have gradually come to respect themselves in their research roles and to be respected by others as well, the way has been paved for expanded research staffing and facilities. The experiences of two investigators who have participated in the growth of research at their institutions may be cited as examples. One respondent, who had had considerable research experience on the East Coast, moved to a Western university psychiatry department with no research facilities and almost no investigative work:

> Our first laboratory was a space previously used for a coal bin, abandoned since they had gone to furnace oil. I had no research money; I set up and equipped it by my own labors, scrounging war surplus, and so on. During this time I acquired a great deal of direct experience with the technical, caretaking, and other aspects of research that have later proven quite valuable. Meanwhile my salary consisted of whatever odds and ends [the department chairman] was able to pull together, supplemented by some consulting at the Veterans Administration Hospital and a small amount of private practice. Trying to get much research time under these arrangements proved a rather frenetic task. The availability of federal stipends to support full-time research involvement was our salvation.
> [Another researcher in the department] extended his research commitment parallel to mine and, by the time we moved to the new medical center, we had sufficient research in progress and sufficient leverage within the power structure of the medical school to be

awarded relatively generous amounts of research space in the new departmental area. . . . The federal support has obviously meant a great deal to me as well as provided a real forward thrust to the department's research growth.

Another psychiatric researcher at an East Coast medical center described a similar growth pattern, although in this instance financial support came from other sources as well:

> Although the Department of Psychiatry [at my institution] had a reputation for being research oriented—a justifiable one considering its past history—at the time I finished my residency in 1955 there was not one person in full-time psychiatric research in the department. What research was on-going was carried out in the context of other duties and was principally, if not entirely, of a clinical nature. In 1957 or 1958 we were approached by a pharmaceutical manufacturer who was interested in forming a relationship with us to establish some basic research as well as to develop a clinical psychopharmacology unit. Since I had expressed a strong interest in research, I was approached by . . . the chairman to take over the development of the program. Nonetheless, the orientation in this department was such that I was not offered a full-time appointment, even though funds were available. Within a short time I managed to recruit two full-time Ph.D. basic scientists (both of whom have since developed their own laboratories and have outstanding scientific reputations). With the success of this development and my own somewhat increased stature in the department, I was able to convince the [department] chairman that I, too, should be a full-time faculty member—probably the first full-time research M.D. in the department. This agreement was to some extent predicated on my ability to obtain support from the Research Development Program and so I duly submitted an application. . . . One of the principal objectives of the program, as I understand it, was to free investigators from other responsibilities so they could do research. In my case that was really followed to the letter. [The department chairman] gave me free rein to develop a research program, never once asking me to do anything that materially interfered. I must say that I think he was impressed with my ability to get the career grant, because he assumed from then on that I would be able to develop and find support for any research that was done in the department.
>  . . . I feel that I have made some contributions to the field and to the department. My research group has grown to include more than 25 doctoral-level scientists.

*Problems of Research Participation.* Despite the many benefits the Research Development Program offers, a number of grantees have had to make significant sacrifices to participate in it. The most obvious sacrifice has been financial. Although the rules of the program were designed to make it possible for an individual to undertake a research career without making a large personal financial sacrifice (see Chapter 6: History of the Research Development Program), it has not worked out that way. As one investigator cited from experience:

> In terms of income, continuing with the Research Career Award has been a significant limitation. Other faculty members on a geographic full-time basis earned considerably more than I did during these years; however, this has been less painful than it otherwise would have been had my wife not been a physician and worked at least part time over most of these years. Accordingly she deserves a considerable amount of the credit for my being able to pursue research and academic work.

For the most part, the researchers appear either to have accepted the financial limitations or to believe that other benefits outweigh this disadvantage:

> The [Research Development Program award] . . . meant forsaking an appealing and comfortable private practice but the satisfaction I derive from my work in neuroscience, the rewards of taking and giving at a scholastic level, [and] my independence in thinking and doing all certainly outweigh the possible financial benefits that I might have obtained from strictly clinical work.

Others have rationalized the program's limitation on private practice as ultimately benefiting their research career:

> I must admit, however, that there were times when I turned down opportunities to do highly remunerative consultations with patients; then I felt some momentary resentment about the restrictions imposed by the program. In all objectivity, however, I think it was a wise proviso to forbid private practice, since it is very easy to get diverted into heavy clinical responsibilities that inevitably detract from one's ability to do research.

*Funding Insecurity.* Although most of the grantees appear to have made peace with their current financial and professional status, for many the future looks less optimistic. The primary problem is that the "seed money" concept on which the program was predicated has not been successful in encouraging academic institutions to assume ultimate financial responsibility for their research faculty members. If anything, it may even have encouraged them to avoid responsibility, since the federal government has assumed such a large share of the financial burden. But times, administrations, and budgets have changed over the past 20 years, and the federal role in research funding is diminishing. Even Research Development Program researchers—who are in a relatively more stable position financially than co-workers who survive with only short-term grants—are justifiably concerned about the future:

> Moral support from the chairman and other members of the department was abundant, but there was a tacit understanding that we researchers would make it on our own as far as financial support was concerned. This dissociation of responsibility for support of research people was fostered by the fact that my salary came from a source outside of the institution. It was a price we were all willing to pay, back then, and it probably was an advantage to the development of our research program because of the opportunities that we had to pursue our research interests unimpeded. However, in more recent years of tight money, we have had to restructure our relationships with the department and to point out that the research function of the department is as integral as the service and teaching [functions]. (This was, of course, the official philosophy and, in fact, the sincere belief of the [department] chairman and the clinical members. However, since the research was self-supporting, there was no necessity to put the theory into practice.) Inter-relationships with the clinical faculty are still being developed, not without some stress and strain, although this department is probably better than almost any I know in this regard. It is simply that it has become necessary for the school to begin thinking about taking on support of research at a time when money for all functions is more difficult to come by.

According to another grantee, anxiety about the future of support for psychiatric research has already taken its toll in the scientific community as some individuals have sought greater security:

> The federal support has obviously meant a great deal to me; however, there have been a number of anxieties that have become more acute in recent years. These relate particularly to the instability and threats to federal programs like the Research Career Awards and the possibility that the next five-year renewal will not occur. This is a particular threat because the medical school simply does not have the funds to carry my salary should federal support not be forthcoming. I suspect that this might be a consideration of some of the research scientists who have opted not to continue on federal support. They may figure that if there is a likelihood of their having to find alternative means of support through practice [or] clinic work, it is better to start this sooner as an option than being forced to do so later by necessity.

Many of the respondents implied or stated outright that the special virtue of the Research Development Program is its relatively long-term support for the individual. The threat of shortened support defeats in many respects the program's intent. As one grantee put it:

> Of course, key to the security offered by the Career Award is the fact that at NIMH one can count on it for a lengthy period, up to 20 years or so. Were the awards to be for a total of only five to seven years, they would offer no more security than any other type of faculty position.

Another investigator felt that even 15 years of support can be inadequate:

> If I should be lucky enough to continue in this program, my eligibility will expire when I am 57. This is too young to quit and too old to start a new career, especially after spending a lifetime crawling farther and farther out on the limb of super-specialization. As a matter of fact, this consideration alone would be enough to keep me from entering the laboratory full-time more than briefly.

Another research scientist also addressed the problem of what he called "re-entry" once one leaves the program:

> Research Development Program awardees at some point face the problem of re-entry into full-time academic life. Assurances about positions cannot, unfortunately, always be implemented in times of tight budgets and cut-backs. In addition, considerable reallocation of time and effort are required in this transition. I believe that a review of such problems undertaken jointly by the administrative staff of the division and by present and former awardees may be helpful.

An awardee who describes himself as being in a basic science area and functioning much more as a physiological psychologist than a psychiatrist summarizes his experience:

> The award has meant to me the opportunity to pursue some answers to questions without distractions from excessive hours of administration, practice, and teaching. The program has enabled me to pursue these matters with colleagues across the land and students locally, developing one experimental pursuit, which, even in the words of my severest critic, is "potentially very fruitful."

Like the awardee cited above, another conducting basic studies believes that the program's ultimate value to himself and others is to contribute vitally needed scientific information to the field of psychiatry:

I am not the one to judge the benefits that others may have received from my work as an awardee, but I have never felt more self-confident than I now feel, never more convinced of the value and relevance of brain research for building a solid framework of psychiatric science. . . . Unquestionably, brain science has made great progress in the past few years. Although this progress has not yet led to dramatic therapeutic breakthroughs, it is precious nonetheless. Because it is scientific, it will not be undone by fads or fancies, and it is most assuredly increasing our knowledge of the brain-mind relations. This is, in my view, a sure way to success in our field, and this is why I love working with my monkeys. The relevance of this work is clear enough to me and to most of my fellow psychiatrists. It may not be clear to the layman, to the taxpayer, or the Congressman who support this work, but if I were asked, I think I would know how to defend it.

How does one assess the impact of an innovative venture such as the Research Development Program? One can talk quantitatively about numbers of grantees, dollars spent, and research papers published. One can also cite trends in the numbers of psychiatrists conducting research on a full-time basis. Yet these statistics fail to communicate the qualitative differences that long-term, career-oriented salary support can make in the life of an individual researcher, especially a psychiatrist. In many instances, it has spelled the difference between trivial research participation and a career essentially devoted to full-time research. For example, many individuals with the interest in and capability for a major commitment and contribution to psychiatric research would have hesitated to choose a full-time research career because security and status in conventional psychiatry departments usually reward the clinician, not the researcher. Support by the Research Development Program has given many potential research scientists the courage to "buck the reward system" and even to change it by their presence in clinical settings. It has also affected the social and professional interactions—both productive and stressful—between program participants and others in their institutional settings. Further, the program has given grantees the freedom to explore problems on a relatively long-term basis, unencumbered by administrative and other distractions or the need for frequent grantsmanship. The high quality and often novel directions of their research reflect this freedom.

## The Behavioral Scientist Researcher

Psychiatric research, considered as a whole spectrum of investigative approaches, depends on the biological, psychological, and social sciences for both substance and technique. A psychiatric problem, in fact, is one that requires a special application of behavioral science, and most psychiatric problems (of development, depression, or drug abuse, for example) have implications for several behavioral sciences. Thus, establishing a scientific basis for psychiatry and improving clinical practice requires that the methods, models, and substantive findings of the behavioral sciences be made available to the community of psychiatric students, practitioners, and researchers. Although there are many possible ways of accomplishing this, one method stimulated by the Research Development Program has been to encourage nonpsychiatrists to conduct their research in clinically oriented psychiatric settings such as the psychiatric departments of medical schools or in their teaching and research hospitals, clinics, and related facilities.

How do nonpsychiatrists use their research competence in non-experimental activities, such as teaching and consultation? Do they find their professional positions more rewarding than conventional positions in their own disciplines? To what extent do they serve as a bridge between psychiatry and their own scientific disciplines?

To find out how working as an "alien" in psychiatric settings has affected these scientists, Dr. Boothe surveyed 24 nonpsychiatric Research Development Program grantees (psychologists, sociologists, biologists) working in such environments. In an open-ended part of the request, respondents were asked to discuss three key issues:

1. *The educational function of the behavioral scientist.*[1] Grantees were asked to explain what they believed their function should be, to describe their own experience, and to explore how and why their own function may have differed from their ideal.

2. *Interdisciplinary relations in psychiatric research.* Respondents were asked to describe how the relationship with other disciplines actually works in a psychiatric department. Both those who enjoyed "productive collaboration" and those who did not were encouraged to comment on their experiences.

3. *The psychiatric setting as an environment for a research career in the behavioral and biobehavioral sciences.* This issue was entirely open-ended, and no suggestions were given as to the types of information sought.

The rest of this chapter will examine replies by 24 respondents (19 psychologists, 2 sociologists, a social psychologist, a neurobiologist, and a neurochemist). Since the sample is small, no attempt will be made to treat these replies statistically. Since the emphasis is on the quality of individual experiences, quotations from respondents will be used extensively.

---

[1] Scientific psychiatry is a behavioral science. However, in this chapter we have narrowed the definition of behavioral scientists to refer to Ph.D.s in disciplines other than psychiatry who work in the psychiatric setting.

### The Educational Function of the Behavioral Scientist

The primary educational function of a behavioral scientist in a psychiatric setting, according to the respondents, is to contribute the special knowledge, skills, and attitudes that differentiate him from most psychiatrists. Typically, this is seen as exposing those who are essentially nonscientists (whether staff or trainees) to the rigorous methodology and intellectual discipline of the research scientist. Education may take many forms. The scientist's special contributions may include teaching or consulting on research methodology or statistics, exposing others to scientific values and research attitudes, or presenting the special knowledge and skills represented by his own particular discipline.

*The Scientist as a Resource Person.* The respondents tended to see themselves (and to be seen by others) as experts in research methods who can help psychiatrists design, conduct, and consume research more rigorously, intelligently, and critically. More than half (13) of the respondents specifically mentioned this role, which one psychologist termed "serving as a resource person":

> The behavioral scientist serves as resource person for the design, analysis, and interpretation of research on etiology, classification, impairment, intervention, and change in child and adult psychopathology. He and his scientist colleagues are often the only persons in the psychiatric setting with training and successful experience in these areas.
>
> He attempts to relate methods, data, and interpretations associated with experimental statistics or other scientific analyses of human and animal behavior and physiology to problems in clinical psychiatry, neurology, and medicine.

The educational role of behavioral scientists may be formal or informal, but the informal contacts (whether with staff, residents, or students) seemed generally to be more satisfactory. A physiological psychologist stated what seemed to be a common experience:

> ... My own image of educational function has changed over the years, and although for a long time I felt I was really not participating in education, in retrospect I find that merely my availability as a behavioral scientist consultant on ways to approach problems of research is, to young faculty members and residents, reason enough for my being a part of the psychiatric setting.

In addition to being a technical resource, a related and to many respondents an equally important educational function of the behavioral researcher is to stimulate rigorous, critical thinking and an open-minded awareness of alternatives. These values were seen by many informants as useful for the future clinician as well as for potential researchers, since the well-informed practitioner needs to learn how to be a discriminating consumer of research information. Of the eight respondents who mentioned the importance of teaching scientific values and attitudes, several mentioned the tendency of psychiatrists (young and old) to accept ideas uncritically, on authority. The nonpsychiatrists frequently alluded to the different thought and behavior styles of the scientist-psychologist-researcher and the physician-psychiatrist-healer and felt that they could at least help to bridge the gap between them. As one psychoanalytically trained psychologist observed:

> ... It seems to me that there are very real differences in the thinking styles of behavioral scientists and psychiatrists (with the former more conceptual, more data-oriented, less absorbed by immediate issues of patient care, and more directed inward to the institution rather than outward to private practice). . . .

Bridging the gap between the disciplines can sometimes require special training and/or effort. The same psychologist continued:

> Much of my personal impact comes because I'm psychoanalytically trained and, to that degree, am less of a foreign body to many of my psychiatrist colleagues. Many of the behavioral scientists here have little or no apparent impact on education (of students or of their colleagues); the gap is wide and characterized by peaceful coexistence.

Many of the themes discussed earlier emerge in the following comments by a comparative psychologist:

> Medical practice demands a well-defined set of skills, the training for which, when overemphasized, may easily lead to the stance that all the required knowledge is already available for practicing the profession. Furthermore, in medical education there is a necessary emphasis on the effective use of authority that, when excessive, may lead to a stance of appeal to authority. In psychiatric education, these factors are further complicated by the emphasis on the use of subjective inference in therapeutic interaction, which also may become excessive, and, when compounded with emphasis on authority and existing . . . skills, may interfere with critical examination of objectively observable information. In light of these, the primary . . . function of research education in a psychiatric setting is the representation of basic scientific values, namely:
>     1. the emphasis on . . . knowledge rather than on the professor

of knowledge (the former thrives on creative skepticism and scientific openness, the latter is threatened by it); and

2. that clinical interaction (whether individual, institutional, or preventive-social) need not and cannot be separated from scientific openness and awareness of the potentialities for individual contribution to knowledge.

The visibility and practice of such values in [the] psychiatric educational setting is essential for all trainees, regardless of their plans for future professional investment in clinical, academic, or research settings. Furthermore, only through direct visibility of these values and through familiarity with styles and approaches of research could a psychiatric trainee with potential talent for scientific contribution fully understand what science is about and apply himself to useful scientific aims. . . .

Another respondent, in discussing the role of the behavioral scientist as educator in the ways of science, raised some more specific points about the lessons to be taught:

Since one rarely finds a psychiatrist approaching a research problem with the same knowledge of experimental design, statistical analysis, or testing tools that a Ph.D. trained in behavior science is presumed to have, the most pervasive function of the latter is to introduce and consolidate such habits of thought into psychiatric research. In particular, I have labored to explain the full meaning of experimental control groups to my psychiatric friends doing both human and animal studies. When dealing with serious residents (some only play at research), I have been gratified by their progressive acceptance of rigorous standards. On the other hand, it is difficult to criticize older psychiatrists; one generally bites one's tongue and affects institutional gemütlichkeit.

A second aspect of teaching research attitudes involves cautioning against loose borrowing of behavioral or physiological terms—"extinction," "arousal," "imprinting." Psychiatrists find magic in new words and only with reluctance admit that each must have an operational definition, which cannot be used in a new context without justifying data. I have used the term "model systems" to discuss animal studies in order to emphasize that experimental findings only suggest ways to formulate and examine clinical phenomena: they do not prove clinical interpretations.

Third, the behavioral scientist should provide a continual well of information and/or references in his field for the psychiatrist to feast upon. Without specialized experience, psychiatrists tend to fixate on and quote back to the first behavioral study they come across; sometimes they need to be pushed back into the library to read about alternative interpretations or new complexities in the data.

In all these teaching functions, one must recognize that a psychiatrist needs to find more practical relevance in research than the usual Ph.D. researcher. The latter wants the former to imitate *his* research style and theoretical perspective. This seems neither realistic nor even efficient, since pure research in my opinion needs to be a nearly 100 percent effort. . . .

*Teaching the Biobehavioral Sciences.*   Some of the respondents viewed themselves and their educational role not only as representatives of the scientific approach in general, but of their own specific disciplines. Thus, they felt that their own disciplinary expertise could and should be shared with psychiatrists who might benefit from it. For example, a neurobiologist has suggested the following role for a biological scientist in the psychiatric setting:

> His or her research should be concerned with basic mechanisms of normal and abnormal nervous function at both cellular and organismic levels, and he or she should be able to discuss [in] (seminars) some of these research findings with colleagues who are looking at clinical aspects of mental function. I consider this intercommunication a most vital part of the role of a neurobiologist in a psychiatric setting. He or she should also collaborate with colleagues in clinical research to investigate nervous function at the human level.

A sociologist has viewed her educational contribution as fourfold. First, she serves as an educator in research methodology (encouraging the use of control subjects and research in nonpatient populations, increasing the reproducibility of research methods by spelling out questions, using nonprofessional interviewers, double-checking coding, testing the reliability of global judgments by psychiatrists, and stimulating the use of computer techniques and the application of more sophisticated statistical methods). She has represented her discipline in other ways:

> [Second,] I have encouraged research at the juncture of psychiatric and social concerns in topics such as education, death rates, criminology, divorce, poverty, ethnic differences, patterns of drinking, and drug use below the level of clear psychopathology; I have reported on findings in these areas from social science literature that psychiatrists do not usually read.
> [Third, and] less important from my point of view, I have attempted to represent the sociological viewpoint, trying to keep the psychiatrists abreast of issues and concerns of sociologists, particularly as related to mental health issues.
> There is a fourth function, which . . . is to bring a recognition of the social role of the patient into problems of clinical assessment and management. On occasion I have been able to do this, for example by pointing out that . . . 16-year-old patients *must* be assessed for drug use.

In general, the respondents did not stress their potential contribution to psychiatric education as communicators of substantive information from their respective fields.

However, two respondents did mention that their skills might be better used if they were "programmed into the educational structure itself" so that, among other benefits, substantive information might be more profitably conveyed. Thus, a psychologist suggested the following:

> I think that behavioral scientists should have a greater role in the formal education of psychiatrists. . . . There are several possibilities. As Skinner and others have observed, there is a considerable amount of learning during psychotherapy, with the psychiatrist often consciously or unconsciously shaping the patient's behavior. Since this is probably unavoidable, psychiatrists might profit from didactic courses on the principles of learning and reinforcement. I'm also optimistic about the possibility of shaping certain types of behavior such as self-assertion or the recognition and expression of feelings in children with emotional problems. Such an approach might lay the groundwork for effective prophylactic psychiatric treatment.

According to one psychologist, if behavioral scientists were included in the educational curriculum of psychiatry, as they are in the medical school itself, he and other psychologists might be viewed as members of one of the sub-specialties in the psychiatry program (such as the sub-specialty of child psychiatry or geriatric psychiatry) rather than as methodological consultants.

In other words, psychology is now treated in many medical schools as a "basic science" (like anatomy or physiology) and taught during the first two pre-clinical years. However, many psychiatric residents attend medical schools in which psychology is not taught (and many have no psychology courses in their undergraduate pre-medical curriculum); such residents might benefit from courses in the theoretical and experimental substance of psychology.

*Communicating Research Relevance.* Several of the respondents, speaking of their interdisciplinary educational role, acknowledged some impediments to communication. Many felt that although their technical contributions were appreciated, they and their research concerns were too often viewed as irrelevant by the clinically oriented psychiatrist, whether staff member or trainee. Yet the continuing confrontations and efforts to bridge this interdisciplinary gap have often brought rewards to those on both sides; clinician and scientist alike have been enriched and their perspectives broadened. As a psychologist put it:

The scientist practicing and teaching in a psychiatric setting is exposed daily to immediate and real mental health demands of individuals and society. In such an atmosphere, if he is worth his salt, he cannot escape into a remote corner of scientific purity: he is forced to consider and explain the relevance of his research to general mental health needs and concerns.

*Teaching Residents.* Many of the respondents distinguished among the many types of students they encountered—medical, graduate, research fellow, staff member, resident—and generally preferred to teach either those in their own discipline or young faculty members. A common complaint concerned residents as students. According to several respondents, these extremely busy psychiatrist-trainees generally have neither the time nor the inclination to become seriously interested in research. Their primary concerns are pragmatic and clinical, and even those who say they are interested in research rarely have the time or patience for the long, drawn-out research process, whether it be clinical or laboratory research. Thus, as one investigator said, "teaching residents is often a thankless job!"

An experimental psychologist discussed some of the problems of teaching young psychiatrists to do research:

> Research training can only be conducted effectively in the laboratory. While formal courses are often necessary prerequisites to the study of many problems, neither the psychiatrist nor anyone else can learn to do research in the classroom. The potential researcher must therefore get into a laboratory and be given enough time and money to accomplish something. Unhappily, in my experience, very few psychiatrists seem to have sufficient time or interest. Their clinical work and other responsibilities seem to come first, and often research is something they feel they might do between lunch and an afternoon round of meetings. . . .
>
> If we are seriously interested in research training, the young psychiatrist must be given at least a year of free mornings or afternoons so that he can be in the laboratory several days per week. Without a prolonged, obligation-free period during which the psychiatrist conducts his own experiment, analyzes his own data, and hopefully, reports his own results, little can be accomplished. Research is a serious and time-consuming occupation. The sooner the student learns this the better, [because] those who do not know what research involves should not dabble in it.

The psychologist's insistence on intellectual skepticism often conflicts with the resident's need for certainty and conviction. Behavioral science, which can thus disrupt the learning of an ideology that will buttress and sustain those who are in a difficult clinical role, is often actively avoided by residents, not just ignored or passed over.

A developmental psychologist who has grappled with the problems of teaching residents has come up with a *modus vivendi* based on his understanding of the resident's point of view:

> Seminar teaching of research to psychiatrists or residents who have not already committed themselves to research has been frustrating and not very effective. Particularly with the residents, the feeling is one of assault. They say, "I'm trying to learn clinical skills, I feel uncertain of myself; your world is too distant from my interests and is, in fact, a threat because I am looking for certainty and authority and you preach doubt and skepticism."
>
> I have found other teaching with residents to be effective and completely gratifying to me and, I think, to them. The ground rules for success are as follows: (1) it must be voluntary participation—entirely elective with no great external pressures to participate; (2) if possible, it is best for the students to choose the topics for discussion and then seek out the faculty member who is best qualified to cover that topic; (3) for content, I've found the relationship of theory to clinical data to be one of the best topics. Thus, rather than being an end in itself, research is brought in almost incidentally as a tool that must be understood.

This apparently successful approach was based on viewing the resident primarily as a consumer rather than as a producer of research information. For the most part, the respondents did not discuss their teaching role with students from their own disciplines, although some appeared to miss serving as a role model for graduate students—their "intellectual heirs." Most seemed to assume that young physicians in departments of psychiatry would choose psychiatrists, not psychologists, as mentors, even if the trainees were research oriented.

## Interdisciplinary Relations in Psychiatric Research

According to these behavioral scientists, their presence in departments of psychiatry frequently meant that they not only taught psychiatrists, but also collaborated with them in conducting research. In the main, these collaborative efforts were regarded as very successful and rewarding. Of the 24 respondents, 14 reported very satisfactory collaboration, while another six reported that their experiences had been a mixture of good and bad. Only two had negative experiences. Of the remaining two, one had no collaborative experience, and the other, while stating that "productive collaboration is essential" did not indicate his own experience.

*Conditions for Successful Collaboration.* Among the factors that contribute to successful collaboration, the respondents frequently cited: compatible personalities of the collaborators, physical proximity and a chance to exchange ideas informally, interest in a common problem and a similarity of outlook, and sufficiently clear distribution of labor and authority to allow each to use his particular expertise to best advantage. The following quotations from grantees will explore some of these points in greater detail.

An experimental psychologist whose collaborative experiences have been very satisfactory noted:

> If there is one good reason for a behavioral scientist to join a psychiatry department, it is the opportunity to participate in interdisciplinary research, not only with psychiatrists and clinicians, but with other biomedical students. Only psychiatry departments seem to offer both sufficient facilities and interested staff personnel (neurochemists, neurophysiologists, neuropharmacologists, and others). My own relationships in this area have been very good, and I have published several papers that could not have been written without the collaboration of people in other disciplines. Indeed, my own research has moved from strictly behavioral to both behavioral and neuropharmacological.

This researcher specified some of the conditions required for successful interdisciplinary efforts:

1. The physical proximity of the laboratories involved (they should be in the same wing or at least the same building);
2. Similar academic rank, position, prestige, and interests of the several investigators;
3. A strong but demanding leader who treats his colleagues as equals, not as technicians;
4. Sufficient time, space, equipment, and job security (it usually takes me three to four years to form a profitable collaboration with another scientist).

Another psychologist, who has observed the collaborative efforts of other psychologists in his department but has not collaborated himself, had the following observations:

> To the extent that some members of an interdisciplinary group are more equal than other members of the group, one does not have an interdisciplinary setting but [instead] one investigator who heads a team of very high-level technicians. I am not advocating research by majority vote, but I am not willing to dignify a group of researchers by labeling it a multidisciplinary team simply because the

members may come from different fields. Interdisciplinary research must evolve from a common interest rather than be the result of a technical necessity. In other words, there must be a conceptual input from the very beginning—there must be real communication and mutual respect.

The [way] the relationships between different behavioral scientists evolve and work is probably as varied as the number of settings in which such groups exist. In my view, the success of any such group is based on the personal interactions among the members of the group and not on any administrative structure that may be devised.

Like several others, another psychologist stressed the importance of the personalities and research interests—rather than the disciplines—involved in collaboration:

As investigators mature, the identification with a particular discipline becomes weaker and weaker. One has a problem to solve or a set of problems, and any techniques—no matter from what discipline they are derived—become fair game. To me the whole concept of disciplines is for the convenience of the training and licensing institutions. From what I've seen, it has relatively little influence in research. I've known some people for several years through our interest in common problems only to find out later that somebody I've assumed to be a psychiatrist is a psychologist, or vice versa. Our psychiatry department may be unusual in this regard, but of all the conflicts and difficulties that have emerged over the years, those associated with professional identification have been the least important. Collaboration is another problem. By and large I feel it has less to do with [one's] discipline than with individual personality. I've worked with one psychiatrist for over 15 years with almost no problems—or rather, with no major problems that couldn't be worked out. I can't say the same for some psychologists with whom I've collaborated.

*Division of Labor.* Although disciplines may matter little in the success of these collaborative arrangements, there is often a division of labor along disciplinary lines among interdisciplinary collaborators, with the behavioral scientists contributing research techniques and methodological skills, while the psychiatrists provide clinical knowledge, access to appropriate patients, and patient management:

I have enjoyed happy and productive collaboration with the psychiatrists in our department. We complement each other. They provide clinical know-how and I provide technical and methodological skills. There has been a very open and generous giving of help, even when active collaboration on the same project is not involved.

Some variations on the same theme were mentioned, as typified by the following comments by a sociologist, but even in this example the division of labor is essentially conventional:

> We have not had a feeling of being interdisciplinary in the sense that psychiatrists and I contributed very different things to the research or roped off special domains. We each brought questions that we wanted answered to the research and these probably differ somewhat according to our disciplines. There are certain areas in which psychiatrists have total responsibility—for example, in making diagnoses. The way they normally ask symptom questions during a psychiatric evaluation is used as the model by which to construct standard questionnaires that could be used by laymen. They also were relied on to go over questionnaires with lay interviewers to train them to ask the psychiatric questions. Interviewers are taught to act like psychiatrists in asking questions—that is, to act as though the questions come out of their own interest, not just mechanically off the page. Psychiatrists also provide access to patient groups and patients to be used for pre-testing and training lay interviewers and subjects. My own role as social scientist is predominantly in designing the continuity of interviews, their format, selecting interviewers, designing codes, and planning and carrying out the analysis. Writing, in principle, is shared, but I tend to take the heavier responsibility because I usually end up being more familiar with the data and how it was analyzed. However, sometimes the psychiatrist takes the responsibility for a first draft, and I play the role of critic-reviser. . . .

Occasionally, there is a dramatic disciplinary role reversal, as in the following example cited by a psychoanalytically trained psychologist:

> An example of more unusual collaboration is the development of a joint project on behavioral treatment approaches to essential hypertension. I'm working in the development of this project with . . . [Dr. X], a nationally recognized research person in behavior therapy and a psychiatrist, [and Dr. Y], a psychoanalyst who is outstanding in his inventiveness for development of [measuring] devices. . . . All three of us are experienced behavioral scientists. My special contribution, however, is in the design of the research, although it is certainly not my unique contribution. [Dr. X's] contribution is in the suggestion of behavioral treatments. [Dr. Y's] is in measurement devices. This certainly is different from the "common-sense" clichés about interdisciplinary approaches to psychiatric problems, since I, as a behavioral scientist (but also a psychoanalyst), am also contributing on the level of clinical sophistication. [Dr. X], who is a psychiatrist, is contributing on the level of behavior therapy techniques (most usually in the realm of the

psychologist). [Dr. Y], a psychoanalyst, is contributing on the level of equipment sophistication as well as the more usual clinical awareness of the meaning of our procedures to the patient.

At the organizational level, behavioral scientists often feel that collaborative efforts work best when they are in positions of senior authority or when they are decisively responsible for design and methodological aspects of the research. A clinical psychologist reported that under these conditions, his collaboration with clinicians generally goes reasonably well:

> ... so well, in fact, that I don't think they or I conceive of the work as interdisciplinary in character. In another sense these clinical experiments do not raise some of the common problems of interdisciplinary research. They are not, strictly speaking, collaboration between two experienced investigators. I am clearly identified as the senior research person, while my collaborators include those who are clearly identified as the clinicians responsible for the clinical management aspects of the research itself.

Another psychologist elaborated on the division of responsibility he sees as important for constructive collaboration:

> I have found interdisciplinary cooperation quite rewarding and useful. I think that my own experience in this is partly determined by the fact that I enter into such collaboration only when I am assured that I have some say both in the development of the problem and in the manner that the problem will be attacked. I learned to do this several years ago, after a few very unfruitful collaborations (not fruitful from my point of view, although apparently more successful from the point of view of others) in which the problem of who shares control was both undefined and unsatisfactory. The issue here is not that of a power struggle *per se*, but rather of educating psychiatrists to recognize the necessity for nonpsychiatrists to have decisive power in those areas of the problem where they are expected to make the most contribution. . . . Psychiatrists very often have an imperialistic attitude and therefore tend to structure things in a very hierarchical fashion. Being trained in medical school to have absolute (life-and-death) responsibility, they carry with them the wish for absolute control.

The respondents have generally found it easier to collaborate with younger psychiatrists and residents than with senior members of the department. As one psychologist observed:

> In my own department there is little collaboration between high-ranking peers. Most of the collaborative research that exists is carried on among lower ranking members of the faculty.

Another respondent made a similar observation:

> I have profited from research collaboration with younger psychia-
> trists and residents. The older men have been less interested (some
> outright opposed) to systematic research in practical psychiatric
> problems. . . . Such collaboration [as I have had] has been too rare,
> I think; relatively few in this setting have been interested in par-
> ticipating. In part, perhaps, this is because I have had little basis
> for contacting residents and young physicians.

Residents have not always proved to be cooperative collaborators,
however. As one investigator noted:

> There has not been much active collaboration with residents.
> This may be a selection factor. The staff psychiatrists have already
> opted for an academic career that involves interest in research. The
> residents are more representative of psychiatrists at large—that is,
> not so interested in the basic scientific foundations of their art.

This researcher suggested that, given needed changes in the
psychiatric curricula, psychiatric residents of the future may be more receptive to behavioral science research and its practitioners:

> With research becoming more interdisciplinary, psychiatrists are
> in a very favorable position to assume a basic science role. But we
> need some fundamental changes in the conception of what a psy-
> chiatrist is. This will require courage and vision among those who
> make psychiatric curricula. If and when such changes do come
> about, the role of the nonpsychiatrist basic scientist will become
> even more important.

*Problems of Collaboration.*   Although most of the respondents
have been essentially satisfied with their interdisciplinary research efforts,
as noted earlier, six regarded their experiences with mixed feelings. One
cited the inherent strain of tempering individuality in a collaborative
venture:

> I have conducted collaborative research on several occasions.
> These experiences have been some of the most rewarding and most
> painful of my career. The problems that arise in interdisciplinary
> research in psychiatry or in other fields stem in part from a conflict
> within the individual scientist, who must choose between pursuing
> his own interests or partially suppressing his individuality so that
> it conforms to the goals of the group. I believe this is one reason
> why I have seen so many collaborative groups dissolve before they
> have achieved their goals.

A reason for unsuccessful collaboration commonly cited by the grantees has been the lack of sufficient time for their clinical co-workers to participate in the planning of research. For example, a physiological psychologist, who remarked that in the almost nine years of his Career Award he had collaborated effectively and productively with a number of psychiatrists, nonetheless observed that:

> At times the collaborative attempt did not work out satisfactorily because there was no real meeting of the minds and because we didn't take the trouble to hash out all the issues (research and otherwise) involved. The problem rests primarily with the psychiatrists who are too busy with active commitments to be able to sit around for the hours necessary to resolve problems and decide on appropriate methods of research.

A sociologist has had a similar experience in which inadequate time and the difficulties of interdisciplinary communication hampered collaboration:

> The extent of my successful interdisciplinary research is limited; in fact, really long-term collaboration has extended only as far as one social psychologist! And I'm not certain that I would be able to collaborate on a large project with most research psychiatrists without feeling that the quality of the work was in question. This feeling comes from having worked on a number of smaller research projects with psychiatrists and social workers; in these cases there was never enough time to work through the research decisions to the point where everyone felt satisfied with them. The problem occurs in two areas: varied concerns with the importance of specifying the underlying theory; and varied knowledge of and experience with methods of research. I've found that so much time is spent on teaching others and on talking past each other about theory that not much gets done. . . . I think the model must be one in which each person works in his area of competence, contributing his skills, so that [each one's] competence doesn't get watered down by the demands of other specialists. This model is difficult to follow, I think, because much energy must go into making the decisions that allocate certain aspects of the work to each specialist.

Another behavioral scientist has found many aspects of interdisciplinary collaboration difficult:

> Despite the obvious fact that psychopathology, for example, is multifaceted, multidisciplinary approaches to its analysis have not been notably successful. Some reasons may be the following:
> 1. It is difficult, if not impossible, to translate from one discipline

to another, especially when the two disciplines investigate different levels of a system—for example, neural functioning and molar behavior.

2. Multidisciplinary approaches to a common problem tend to get "locked in" to procedures that rapidly become outdated.

3. Few scientists are trained and experienced in more than one discipline. Yet effective cooperation on a cross-disciplinary problem requires more than just communication. It requires that each member of the team be able to conceptualize in the other's field.

4. Multidisciplinary investigation requires new multidisciplinary methods. Few exist, especially for human work.

This investigator also alluded to another problem that has interfered with effective collaboration: failure to understand and see the relevance of one another's fields:

> Most practicing clinicians, though respecting his scholarship, find little of [the behavioral scientist's] discourse to be relevant to their immediate problems. This is unfortunate for both the scientist and his clinical colleagues.

In the case of one psychologist, his lack of collaborative experiences stems directly from his apparent lack of relevance to his more clinically oriented colleagues:

> Most of my own research is with animals and is not of immediate, practical concern to ... potential collaborators. There is, too, the attitude on the part of many clinicians that animal research can contribute little to an understanding of human behavior (unless, of course, it happens to confirm one of their own hypotheses).

A comparative psychologist had dramatically contrasting collaborative experiences: in one setting, there was absolutely no interdisciplinary interaction between researchers, but in his current position he participates extensively in a variety of interdisciplinary efforts. He now distinguishes between two types of interdisciplinary collaboration that he sees as having different likelihoods of success:

> The issue of interdisciplinary collaboration may be broken down into (1) the collaboration of researchers with practicing clinical psychiatrists and (2) the collaboration of a multidisciplinary team of researchers, including, but not exclusively, psychiatric researchers in a psychiatric setting. Though not impossible, there are some serious difficulties with the former. Flexibility of time commitments, freedom for exploring literature, for creative thinking, or for writing

are all indispensable for scientific activity but are rarely available for the practicing clinician who usually works in the tight routine of an eight-hour schedule. On the other hand, the uniform and broad concentration of a psychiatric community on issues of mental health creates an atmosphere of unity in aims, which is, in my opinion, indispensable for multidisciplinary teamwork of researchers.

In all, I feel that due to the necessary mixture of service and training in psychiatric settings, the potentialities for interdisciplinary research are higher [in a psychiatric setting] than in science departments in traditional university settings. In the latter, departmental segmentation, competition for students, tight academic schedules, and so on negatively influence multidisciplinary effort.

When collaborative efforts have been successful, they have often resulted in exploration and information that crosses disciplinary lines and enhances the state of knowledge of all participants, as the following remarks by a neuropsychologist indicate:

In my particular situation, interdisciplinary interactions have been of two kinds: (1) use of an animal model for behavioral pharmacological studies to formulate and test hypotheses about drug effects in man; (2) the use of animal behavioral or electrophysiological paradigms to test biochemical hypotheses. Work on alcohol amnesia in animals, plus my familiarity with experimental literature and human sensorimotor coordination encouraged a collaborative application for research . . . on drug-alcohol interactions in producing deficits in human sensorimotor coordination related to driving skill. In this instance the question about possible potentiation of alcohol effects by drugs commonly prescribed by psychiatrists brings a theoretical question into the realm of medical practice.

Secondly, we view our efforts to dissect out functional neural systems in animals' brains as necessary for detailed testing of hypotheses about molecular mechanisms of drug action. Our institution is unusual in helping to support a substantial laboratory for brain chemistry, but on the whole this work has remained remote from functional analysis of brain or behavior. New opportunities for collaboration arise now that some members are concerned with biochemical effects of biogenic amines or with changes in RNA metabolism that accompany experience. I believe that psychiatric research in basic sciences must be organized around interdisciplinary concepts—"neural and humoral control of aggression" or "biochemical changes in brain relating to depression." Otherwise, such research is better carried out in pharmacology or psychology departments where teaching of specific professional skills can be best achieved.

The Psychiatric Setting as an Environment for a Research
Career in the Behavioral and Biobehavioral Sciences

How adequate is the psychiatric setting for the research career
of a behavioral scientist? Many respondents implied or stated that the
issue cannot be discussed in the abstract; one can assess only how the expectations and qualifications of given investigators (usually themselves)
mesh with the characteristics of the particular psychiatric environments in
which they work. One respondent suggested questions aimed at specifying
aspects of the researcher-environment match:

> 1. Which psychologist? I would venture to say that the person-
> ality characteristics of a research psychologist conducting research
> in a psychiatric or medical setting differ from those of a psychologist
> working in a college of arts and sciences. How independent is he?
> How much does he need feedback from psychologist colleagues?
> What is his attitude toward psychiatrists?
> 2. Which psychiatric setting? Is the psychiatric setting associated
> with the university? Is there any interaction with the department of
> psychology of the university? Is there opportunity to have graduate
> students in the laboratory? What is the commitment of the de-
> partment of psychiatry to the research psychologist? Are there other
> psychologists in the same setting? Why was the psychologist ap-
> pointed to the faculty?
> 3. What kind of research? Are the laboratory facilities available
> in a medical center necessary to implement research? Are collabora-
> tive arrangements necessary or desirable? Are populations of psy-
> chiatric patients necessary for the research? What can this research
> contribute to the research, teaching, and/or service responsibilities
> of the department of psychiatry?
> In summary, the "right" psychologist in the "right" setting doing
> the "right" kind of research would find himself in a supportive
> environment for a research career.

Judging by the responses of those who chose to discuss their
own careers, the ideal meshing of the man, the setting, and the research
is uncommon. For the most part, the respondents commented positively
about their particular setting; 15 stated explicitly that their situation had
been good. Yet eight of those found drawbacks as well, and several alluded
to other colleagues in their disciplines who had not fared as well as they had.

Advantages of the Setting.    The seven whose comments were
completely positive about their experience in the psychiatric setting were
all psychologists; three of them had clinical backgrounds: a clinical psy-

chologist, a psychoanalytically trained psychologist, and a psychologist who was also a psychoanalyst. Most of the others in this group appeared also to share sympathy for and interest in clinical problems.

One of the psychologists, whose research has mostly involved patients in a treatment setting, attributes his success and satisfaction to his clinical research orientation, which may have helped him gain acceptance, status, and salary that other behavioral scientists (either non-clinical or non-research, or both) have not obtained:

> In contrast to the clinical psychologist's [traditional] role, as a researcher I have had as much freedom and support as I felt was appropriate, except for the first few years before I had proven myself as an independent investigator. . . . At present I feel that decisions about who is to be principal investigator on a grant, for example, are made in terms of the specific skills and commitments of the collaborators, and that beyond this my background as a Ph.D. rather than an M.D. is not a consideration either locally or during the grant review process. In my institution the salary differential between M.D.s and Ph.D.s that is evident at lower levels has all but disappeared for me, again in contrast to clinical psychologists, who top out at somewhat lower levels even if they have the top administrative post available to a psychologist.
>
> I think this psychiatric setting can be less hospitable to non-M.D. investigators whose research interests are not in areas obviously applicable to clinical practice. We have a number of them, and they have lab space and reasonable support, but I have heard them say that they are in a poorer position in the institute because they are not doing "relevant" research. I am not convinced that this is really the case, but you can keep in mind that my own views may be related to my areas of research rather than my professional identification. . . .

Many of those who have been enthusiastic about working in the psychiatric setting, regardless of the degree of clinical relevance of their own work, have found it stimulating to be in an atmosphere in which clinical work takes place. Frequently they have cited the reality of having to confront social and psychological problems in a way rarely known to their more conventionally placed academic colleagues. Or, as a social psychologist expressed it, "Relevance is always breathing down your neck." Another researcher elaborated on this point:

> The most enjoyable aspect of the psychiatric setting has been . . . that at least in these settings one has the feeling that research can be focused and directed toward the solution of real problems. In a psychiatric setting there is an appreciation for the fact that sometimes solutions do not come easily nor are answers very clean cut.

This is in contrast to many academic non-psychiatric settings, where the model for research too often tends to be that of the laboratory experiment, where if answers are not easy to come by, then at least the experiment should be clean cut and elegant. For me, the psychiatric setting allows a pursuit of research interests in a manner that is both compatible with my own estimation of what is required for these problems and accepted and facilitated by one's colleagues in the psychiatric field.

A comparative psychologist, who also had highly favorable comments about his experience in a psychiatric setting, specified some of the other stimulating aspects of the environment that have made him prefer it to the university psychology department:

I have chosen this setting in favor of traditional university departments in my field and have found the psychiatric setting beneficial for a research career because: (1) [there is] constant contact with a variety of issues of human behavioral development, and these, I believe, form the overall structure for basic research on general comparative problems of early behavioral development as well; (2) in addition to the rewards of contributing to a field of concentration, there are the rewards of representing a field in the macrocosm of larger mental health concerns and thereby of enriching the latter; (3) growth opportunities and satisfactions are greater in interdisciplinary participation than in narrow concentration and training of specialists in one's own image and field; and (4) a psychiatric setting is highly conducive for professional interaction and provides a variety of ways for participation with issues that expand one's immediate research involvements.

For one behavioral scientist, the experience of working in a psychiatric setting is so rewarding that he is helping now to shift the locus of psychology graduate education from the university to the medical school:

The fact that I've stayed in the same department for 18 years— my entire post-doctoral career—should indicate that basically I've been pleased with it. . . . I like the real-life quality of the medical school in contrast to the more academic departments of psychology. . . .
If we become task-oriented rather than discipline- or self-oriented, then the possibilities of fruitful interchange are almost endless. We are moving more and more of the Ph.D. training in psychology over to the medical school because this is where the action is, both for clinical training and for research.

*Disadvantages of the Psychiatric Setting.*   Many of the respondents with more mixed feelings shared appreciation for the same positive aspects of the psychiatric environment, but found negative aspects of the setting as well. Frequently they felt it to be quite exciting but not very secure. Thus, several found the environment highly stimulating for research and often reported that they were very productive, yet they complained that professional advancement and the acquisition of a tenured position often eluded them. One investigator appeared to accept his professional insecurity relatively stoically, even optimistically:

> I believe I am probably a team man. The psychiatric setting provides all kinds of professions, interests, viewpoints, and skills. In terms of productivity, the setting has been excellent for me. In terms of career advancement, the setting has not been as rewarding in and of itself. But this may be a function of the academic aspects of the entire situation, and not of the fact that it is a psychiatric setting. I have no real reason for complaint. If I had really wanted the tenured professorship, I've had opportunities that I could have taken.
>
> I suspect that academic ladders for behavioral scientists will open up in medical settings more and more, and the Research Development Program has probably helped in that a lot.

Another experimental psychologist found that "formidable if not insurmountable problems" painfully outweighed the many advantages of his position:

> This questionnaire has arrived at a time when I am very seriously considering leaving my position in a department of psychiatry (after 12 years) and joining an academic psychology department. By and large I feel that while I have certainly learned a great deal and have been productive at least as far as my research is concerned (I have more than 52 publications), most psychiatric settings are not the best places for nonclinical scientists to find more or less permanent homes. . . .
>
> First, one has no real identity. The primary functions of a psychiatry department are to train clinicians and to provide clinical services. Research comes third, and most psychiatrists know it. Few medical students or residents have worked in my laboratory over the years and [the] more senior members of the staff tolerate my existence but do not invite me to participate in policy decisions. Moreover, this attitude is reflected in promotions and tenure decisions. After 12 years I am still an Associate Professor and have no tenure. . . .

The problem of loss of identity mentioned above was faced by other respondents as well. A neurophysiological psychologist put the issue trenchantly:

There has been relatively little scientific help or stimulation from my psychiatric colleagues, and I was quite lonely, scientifically speaking, in the early days. It is very important to bring in colleagues and students (via grants and fellowships). It is also urgent to keep in touch with one's field via meetings, study sections (if one is so lucky), and other sources of stimulation. (One should consider implanting pairs of scientists in clinical departments so they can keep each other company.) Colleagues and stimulation are important; without them, one risks feeling out of it professionally and thereby losing one's unique value and identity. To put it crudely, one has to remember what one's interests are and avoid the temptation (or danger) of becoming a half-assed psychiatrist.

Related to the lack of security and sometimes indefinite identity is the frequently-alluded-to problem of being in some respects a second-class citizen in the department:

I don't know to what extent the psychiatric setting has helped or hindered my work. The affiliation with a medical school certainly helps in making contacts with the community (for subjects and so on), and this clearly is a benefit. The focus of a psychiatric department on service also keeps one much more aware of relevant problems. This is in contrast to the often isolated type of work that goes on in academic departments of psychology. On the other hand, the feeling of being a non-M.D. in a medical setting has many well-known disadvantages, and I have felt these as well. I am not sure, however, to what extent the feeling of being a second-class citizen has actually hampered my work.

The feeling of second-class citizenship is sometimes related to antagonism or at least lack of understanding between clinicians and researchers. A psychologist notes that:

The major disadvantage of doing research in a hospital psychiatric setting comes from an antagonism between people engaged in basic research, such as myself, and clinicians. Clinicians feel that there is little room in the hierarchy of the department for people who work chiefly with rat brains. We feel that basic research has contributed significantly to psychiatric therapy and deserves a place in that hierarchy. However, the department is controlled largely by clinicians. Therefore we are almost totally dependent on outside support for our positions in the department.

Another experimental psychologist has also suffered from cross-disciplinary misunderstanding:

My working assumption is that pathological performance of a task depends on the same mechanisms as a normal performance of the same task. In this view, understanding pathological behavior amounts to understanding the mechanism of the behavior (both normal and abnormal) and isolating the parameter(s) whose modification leads to the pathology. Such an assumption minimizes the differences between interests of the clinical and experimental psychologist.

Given this approach, it has been quite appropriate for me to work in a psychiatric setting. I must admit, however, that my clinical colleagues have often viewed my work as if they couldn't believe I really take it seriously. On the other hand, I have sometimes been amazed and baffled by the literal and often unquestioned acceptance of psychiatric lore by some of them. This has made real communication difficult and I have often felt isolated. At the same time, I realize that this is lessening, perhaps in part because I and others like me have shared the psychiatric setting with clinical colleagues.

A clinical psychologist cited several reasons why the psychiatric setting is difficult for research; his thoughts have implications for future directions in education that could overcome these problems:

1. The clinical psychologist usually has no control over patient management unless he is also charged with intervention. Even the research-oriented psychiatrist has considerable difficulty with this because his clinician colleagues, faced with immediate problems of patient management and treatment, cannot usually sustain the slow, scholarly . . . process of clinical or experimental research.

2. The experimentally oriented clinical psychologist usually turns to problems that are peripheral to psychopathology, such as drug research, where he can get better control of the situation.

3. A few clinical psychologists are doing important research in classification, etiology, physiology, intervention, and outcome in psychopathology, but not many. Such operations require too much cooperation and support from too many people.

4. Clinical psychology training programs are not on the mark. Psychologists trained for research usually know little or nothing about clinical problems, the clinical arts, or the management of patients. Many researchers spend their careers working on issues that have only the most tenuous relations to central problems in psychiatry and medicine.

On the other hand, many, if not most clinical-clinical psychologists being trained these days have no training, skill, or experience in the experimental analysis of behavior or in other aspects of scientific psychology.

The scientist-clinician needs to be brought closer to the clinic, and the clinician-clinician should be given more training and experience in research.

In summary, the psychiatric department can prove to be a stimulating and rewarding environment for the behavioral scientist, encouraging extensive interdisciplinary interaction for both teaching and research activities and providing the excitement and humane relevance of a milieu focused on alleviating human suffering. The behavioral scientist is, however, an alien and, even in the best of situations, often experiences some of the hazards of being a scientist and a non-M.D. in a world dominated by clinically oriented physicians: a loss of identity, lack of esteem, and being perceived as irrelevant to the primary concerns of clinical psychiatry. Although some degree of strain appears to be inevitable, it can be minimized if the behavioral scientist has some appreciation of the dominant values of the host department and can communicate to students and staff the relevance of his work to clinical practice. In addition, his own identity can be strengthened by having other scientists like himself in the department or at least readily accessible. He will obviously feel most welcome in a department that encourages and values research sufficiently to reward him in status, security, and salary on a scale commensurate with other departmental members.

# Training for Research

**4**

*The Training Experience*

How does a psychiatrist become a psychiatric researcher? Medical-school training is designed to educate physician-healers; it emphasizes establishing confidence and competence in the healing arts. In its extreme form, such training is the opposite of what would be ideal for producing medical research scientists. In gross outline, medical training exaggerates the distinction between the scientific and the professional points of view to a degree that makes it impossible, at least in Albee's (1970) view, for both presumably antithetical attitudes to exist in one person. Yet with training, many psychiatrists have found a way to retain their professional identity and to become research scientists as well.

One pattern or model for training mental health research workers is to permit young psychiatrists to complete all or the major portion of their medical and specialty training and then to support them in whatever further education is required to make them competent researchers. (For discussion of other approaches, see Chapter 5, "Toward the Future of Psychiatric Science.") The Research Development Program has followed this model in its Type I awards, which have gone primarily to young psychiatrists, providing five years of salary support, funds for special training, and occasional small grants to support the research activities of the candidates. (For further discussion of the various types of awards offered by the program, see Chapter 6.)

Little effort has been made to establish a standard pattern of research training for young psychiatrists. Instead, each candidate has been urged to custom-tailor a program of training to suit his own needs for additional knowledge, methodological background, and research skills.

The only organized training aid offered by the Research Development Program has been support for either annual conferences, which serves to bring together for a brief period all of the investigators holding Type I awards, or for occasional special meetings of investigators working in a common area, such as research on sleep.

There has been a shifting pattern of research training plans over the brief span of the program. For the first five or six years beginning in 1954, a majority of the awardees chose only one method of preparation for psychiatric research: undergoing training in psychoanalysis. During more recent years, this method has appealed infrequently, giving way to a variety of training proposals aimed at skills needed for specific projects, involving various degrees of formal and informal training experiences, and oriented to the basic behavioral sciences. Thus the character of the training plans over the years has reflected the character of the prevailing pattern of research in psychiatry.

Dr. Boothe undertook to determine the character of the training experiences of a small number of grantees preparing to become research workers. He asked them to analyze their own experiences with the training aspects of the program, and he received replies from 15 grantees who had received Type I awards: 13 psychiatrists and two other behavioral scientists. What follows is an analysis of the content of these responses.

*Can a Candidate Plan His Own Research Training?* The answer to this question was generally affirmative. The general experience of this group was that they could foresee what would be needed in the research career they had set for themselves, and they were able both to plan their training and to carry it out successfully. The exceptions to this general assessment were few.

A few candidates found it difficult to anticipate their training needs over a full five years. This group, as well as some of those who thought they had planned the full five years properly, saw their training developing in ways they had not anticipated. Only one man reported that his training plan had been essentially a mistake. He had undertaken psychoanalytic training as the sole preparation for research and ultimately found that in doing so he had failed to prepare himself for the actual research he carried out; he thus assessed his psychoanalytic training as a handicap in his research career.

*Psychiatrists and Behavioral Scientists as Research Trainees.* While there are only two behavioral scientists in the group, the contrast between their training experiences and those of the psychiatrists is clear and probably representative of a much larger group. The behavioral scientists came to the program well trained in research from every point of view. Unlike individuals with prior psychiatric training, they noted no difficulties in acquiring scientific attitudes and methodologies.

However, obtaining clinical experience and contact with clinical material has been difficult for one of the behavioral scientists whose experience is probably not uncommon. To study the problems in which he is interested, he repeatedly felt he needed an M.D. degree. He finds access to patients difficult to obtain without proper credentials.

*Formal Courses.*   Given the extensive formal training many Research Development Program grantees have undergone to achieve an M.D. degree and a specialty in psychiatry, it is notable to find them taking additional formal courses in their research training. A number of investigators have found it useful or even indispensable to take substantive courses over a wide range of subject matter. The courses selected tend to be seminal to the research planned by the investigator; they are courses that seem to have been either unavailable in the medical curriculum or presented in insufficient depth—child development in psychology or genetics, for example.

The training plans of the psychiatrists also show a heavy emphasis on methodological courses—statistics, research design, and the use of computers. These courses have posed various types and degrees of difficulty but have been generally evaluated as ranging from "very useful" to "indispensable."

Many investigators report varied experiences with formal seminars; occasionally they report limited value for formal courses beyond the first one or two. However, most investigators commented quite favorably on ad hoc and self-initiated courses for filling in gaps and keeping up with the latest advances in their fields of interest.

Several of the young psychiatrists argue that the common problems involved in switching from psychiatric practice to psychiatric research would merit three- or four-week crash courses in statistics, methodology, and the values of science for each new crop of awardees.

*Senior Research Sponsors.*   A common element of all training plans is the designation of a senior scientist who is an advisor or consultant. This pairing of a junior and senior investigator appears to have worked well in many instances. When it has not been a functional training device, supervision usually was not needed. Only occasionally has a sponsor been generally unavailable or otherwise remiss in fulfilling his role.

In the ideal case, the senior research consultant-advisor can serve an intense didactic function. One highly productive investigator recounts his difficulties in returning to research after a period of intensive clinical involvement. He says:

> When I went back to tackle the research problem, I still had the darndest time. I felt the seductive pull to retreat to intuitive free-for-all behavioral evaluation techniques. Dr. ———, my sponsor, forever insisted and at times demanded: (1) You must specifically define what behaviors you are following. These must be operationally defined with great care. (2) You must design adequate methods to observe, measure, and record the behavior. Data must be recorded in a form that renders them amenable to statistical analysis. (3) There are such things as control groups. Go get them, and do it with great care. (4) You must be concerned with issues of validity, reliability, and statistical evaluation in behavioral investigations.
> I found this rigidity and discipline the hardest to recapture. My work was much less fun than what I previously did in clinical psychiatry. In fact, much of what I was forced to do was rather boring and repetitious. This was the hardest part for me. But of course it was the most productive.

The research advisors for many of the investigators included individuals who had not been named sponsors for their training. Nearly every investigator mentioned this happening at least once. Sometimes such advisors were formally designated as the research advisor even though they were from another department or discipline.

A very prominent role of the sponsor, whether official or unofficial, is simply that of the model. There appears to be no greater influence in the development of a research investigator than to be in personal contact with someone of extraordinary ability and to watch him deal with moment-to-moment and day-to-day problems. Most of the investigators mentioned this factor in some form.

Finally, senior sponsors have played a very prominent role for these young investigators simply as advisors. Some report that such people had pointed out possibilities that never would have occurred to them unaided. Day-to-day availability of senior research consultants for advice and consultation has been a pervasive element in the development of nearly all of these young mental health Career Investigators.

*Apprenticeship.* A variation on the relationship between a sponsor and a junior investigator is that of apprenticeship. Many junior investigators are too independent at the outset to enjoy an apprentice relationship, but others find this role very productive. While it works very well for some junior investigators, there is a fundamental incompatibility between the apprentice role and the creativity required of the successful research investigator. It is therefore not surprising that the strongest advocates of the apprenticeship system for junior investigators are those who have already undertaken the training of others; they are advocating apprenticeship for their students and not for themselves.

*Learning from Peers.*   A source of instruction and learning mentioned quite frequently is the peer, especially in some other field. One respondent says:

> I have begun a series of collaborative efforts with a group of endocrinologists and psychoendocrinologists and have learned a great deal about hormone systems and biological rhythms.

Another notes that:

> A somewhat unanticipated fallout of my Career Award is the opportunity for almost daily interaction with experimental psychologists. Because of this, my knowledge of research design, data analysis, and other areas has improved considerably.

Still another says:

> I have relied on a wide variety of colleagues for special instruction and consultation.

*Conferences.*   Some aspects of the role of the conference in the research training of investigators are best described by the investigators themselves. The conferences on a special topic tend to have immediate effect. One investigator observed:

> There were many different experiments ranging in topic from physiology to psychology. It gave me an idea of the variety of methods used and contact with relevant people. Also, attending these meetings over two or three years gave me an idea of what kinds of . . . approximations of method to problem might be made.

The annual Career Investigator Conferences, because of their broader range of subject matter and scope, appear to have had both immediate and delayed effects. One investigator notes:

> As global as these . . . meetings were, they brought me involuntarily up against such a wide range of research people that I could

not avoid making meaningful contact with areas close to mine that were utilizing techniques or conceptualizations helpful in my own work. I venture to say that the only real gains I have ever made in understanding the need for statistical analysis of data, adequate research design, and experimental control were accomplished through talking about my work in small group sessions and receiving constructive appraisal.

As another stated:

Although I did not realize its importance to me at the beginning, there was time to see how different types of research problems meshed with different styles of problem solving. The importance of learning the pitfalls and advantages of various methodologies and designs was clear to me after frustrating experiences with my own design problems in the first two years of the award.

*Learning from Students.*   A number of investigators point out how much they have learned from students. A frequent pattern is for a Career Investigator to organize a research team composed of individuals ranging from peers to undergraduate students. Learning from them can be wholly informal, but it occasionally takes a semi-formal turn in the ad hoc, or spontaneous, seminar. In such groups, each person tends to have an area of expertise or unusual knowledge to share with others. For at least one investigator, the role of students as teachers is profound. He writes:

Very important in this respect was the entry into my lab of excellent graduate students undertaking fellowships with me. They opened my eyes to new needs and new techniques. This is my major avenue of growth now.

*Teaching Research.*   Anyone who has ever taught it is aware that in preparing to teach and actually teaching, the teacher learns much more than the student. Many of the investigators have made teaching a part of their full-time research activity, apparently with profit. As one reported:

Another facet of my experience that has added a dimension to training is my teaching research to others. I have several graduate students from the department of psychology in my lab. When required to assess and explain research plans to others, one is constantly forced to evaluate one's own work.

Another says:

> Perhaps the most gratifying of all has been the creative teaching I have had the freedom to pursue. Such teaching has been intimately related to my research.

And, finally, one reports:

> The award also allowed me to become involved in bringing along students at the resident and medical school level. . . . These students have been of extremely high caliber and, as is usual, in teaching one learns so much more than one teaches. I have come to find this form of teaching, which involves intimate work on problems at all levels—from conceptualization and data gathering to re-conceptualization and design of new studies—to be the most rewarding kind of teaching I have ever been involved in.

*Visits to Other Laboratories.* Nearly every investigator has found occasional visits to other laboratories, ranging in duration from a few days to several years, exceptionally valuable and nearly indispensable. Sometimes as long as two years is required to learn another investigator's techniques. The impact of such visits appears to stem from exposure to very different approaches to the same or similar problems. Some of the benefits are apparent from the testimonials of a number of young research psychiatrists:

> A further dimension was added when I began to share and discuss my work with other laboratories. I found that other philosophies and different strategies continually forced me to reassess my own direction and plans.

> The opportunity to visit other laboratories is proving to be a quite useful training experience, perhaps slightly more so than I thought originally. I find it necessary to spend many days at a place in order to benefit from the experience. . . . I am beginning to feel the need to spend a period of time—perhaps four months at another laboratory—to get another perspective and possibly to spend some time doing field or semi-naturalistic observation. . . .

> Currently, I am applying to a private foundation for funds to spend three months with several senior scientists in London. I feel that any scientist should now and then be exposed to the more radical and newer ideas in his field of research. I have found that this can best be done by visits to other laboratories, particularly to the laboratories of the younger up-and-coming scientists. This occasionally can be frustrating, since the innovative nature of some of the work makes it difficult to evaluate before you make your visit,

but I have personally found such visits to be generally quite rewarding. . . .

These visits were valuable in learning of recent developments, although I think that more than two weeks would be required to master some of the techniques.

In terms of learning, visiting other investigators stands out as an enormously rich experience. I learned new techniques and methods and became aware of many new ideas in the field long before their publication in the literature. In addition, I learned how others work—in particular, how they relate prediction to data generation, hypotheses to concepts, concepts to theories, and theories to models. The importance of new models became more and more impressive to me.

I actually carried out my plan to visit other labs for two consecutive summers during the fourth and fifth year of my training, and it was a most productive venture. I am indebted to this very day to the experience of those two summers and still use that training on an almost daily basis.

*The Training Role of Doing Research.* Perhaps the most essential elements that must be stressed in training for research are the strong need to do actual research and the catch-as-catch-can way of acquiring needed information and techniques. One investigator says:

I feel that what is most important is that the researcher have a realistic idea of what areas he needs training in, that he be highly motivated to seek this training, and that a sufficiently large group of scientists be available at his institution so that, whatever his needs entail, he is certain to find an expert with whom he can work.

Other scientists have commented in the same vein:

I do not think I would have absorbed much, however, if I had not been immersed in attempting to carry out some simple projects of my own in my own lab. They served the vital purpose of teaching in precise terms what I did not know. This articulation of one's own ignorance defines exactly what has to be acquired in order to do what one wants to do. . . . In short, I do not think training for research can be sensibly separated from attempting to do research, except for the mastery of one or another limited technique. I would advocate a form of on-the-job training involving aspects of tutorial and apprenticeship, but going beyond either in involving the trainee to train himself as efficiently as possible.

I was given an experimental problem and some general guidelines and essentially put on my own. I developed some techniques and was guided by Dr. ———— and others. The work unfolded as a result.

The kind of training I found most effective was having the time to do my own work and learn by trial and error.

One of the more experienced scientists who responded to this issue is very positive concerning learning by doing and is impatient with formal training for research:

I am very impressed with the self-made man—for example, several recent Nobel Prize recipients. Somehow organizing one's behavior around task accomplishment seems to be much more productive than diffuse preparation for future work. It has been my observation that those who really produce in research learn how to as they do so. I have personally known several recipients of . . . awards who wasted their time thinking about problems rather than actually tackling them. A major aspect of my post-graduate education has been around the practical problems that necessarily have to be solved if the eventual goal is to be realized. Whenever I have stopped the process and tried to educate myself in a broader sense, I have generally found it more of a diversion than a help. Dr. ———— has probably one-tenth of the formal education as a host of "trained" people who are still wondering what to do next.

*Generalities of Research Training.* The policy of allowing applicants for research training to specify their own needs, methods, and patterns of acquiring knowledge has persisted throughout the history of the Research Development Program. Its wisdom is apparent from this account of the experiences of Type I investigators. No curriculum, even in very general form, emerges from examination of the 15 accounts of research training experience.

The most common elements are motivation, stimulation, freedom, and direct research experience. A high level of motivation to do research and the drive and energy required to seek out, learn, and use what is needed is clearly the first requisite. Resources are necessary, but no particular set of resources—be they courses, senior consultants, peers, students, or even visits to other laboratories—is a necessity for everyone. Some sort of stimulation does appear to be necessary. This can be as particular as intensive work with one man, as brief as an annual meeting of a group focused on a narrow set of problems, or as broad and brief as an annual meeting of the broad spectrum of mental health career investigators. What is necessary is some corrective feedback on the individual's own efforts and the broadening influence of examining the efforts of others. Freedom to direct most of one's energies to research appears essential. Freedom to change one's plan when the need for change becomes apparent also seems necessary. One investigator says:

> It seems to me now that one should *train for change* and not simply gamble on one currently fascinating, but narrow, operation. Finally, there appears to be no substitute for doing research as a means of training to do research.

### Psychoanalysis as an Element in Research Training

The dominant role of psychoanalysis in psychiatry in the first half of this century, the almost universal requirement of psychoanalytic training for a career in psychiatric research at the beginning of the Research Development Program (when it was the Career Investigator Grant program), and the clear evidence of recent decline in the dominance of psychoanalysis require that this topic be treated in more depth than other aspects of training for research in psychiatry. Since the pattern appears to be changing very rapidly, let us take an historical approach in explaining the contemporary situation.

*1954–1960.* In the early years of the program, undergoing psychoanalytic training was the dominant mode of research preparation for psychiatrists. Proposals for psychoanalytic training, requests for special training funds to pay for it, and discussion about the function of such training for specific investigators in given lines of research were much more conspicuous in the deliberations of the Selection Committee (the program's advisory body, which provides peer review of prospective candidates and their work) than any other method of adjunctive training for the young investigator, more conspicuous even than all other aspects of training for a research career put together. From 1954 through 1960, of the 18 psychiatrists supported by the Career Development Awards, 16 (or 89 percent) either before or during their involvement in the program had psychoanalytic training. Since members of this group were generally older and more experienced than later candidates, a good share of them came in with psychoanalytic training. Still, one-half of them were funded for psychoanalytic training during the course of their awards. This group of investigators has established an outstanding record in research productivity and has far exceeded the original hopes that one out of three or four of them might become genuine mental health scientists.

The following statement taken from minutes of the Selection

Committee meetings in November 1959 and January 1960 explains the viewpoint of the Committee members and their rather permissive criteria for evaluating proposals for psychoanalytic training:

> Psychoanalytic training may be considered indispensable for one whose research requires data to be obtained by psychoanalytic techniques. Psychoanalysis may also be considered as one desirable source of training for research with clinical phenomena, which requires sensitivity to dynamic processes, personal interaction, and unconscious factors in behavior. Psychoanalytic training may often be regarded as unnecessary . . . for research on purely biological or physiological problems. For some applicants, therefore, psychoanalytic training may be confidently approved as desirable or disapproved as irrelevant. With some applications, however, difficult evaluations must [consider] . . . the applicant's aptitude, his motivation toward clinical research, and the possibility that psychoanalytic training might be an incentive as well as a preparation for clinical research.

Several considerations kept alive the issue of psychoanalytic training. For one, the financial cost was appreciable; for some individuals, it might run to over $5,000 per year, although program policy was to pay not more than three-fourths of the cost to the candidate. A larger cost was in the candidate's time and energy. There was also the recurring question of the relevance of psychoanalytic training to much of the research conducted by grantees.

*1961–1966.* During the next six years, development awards were made to 38 psychiatrists, 25 of whom engaged in psychoanalytic training either before or during the program. Of these, 23 were supported by funds for that purpose under the provisions of the award. Thus the percentage of psychiatrists who had had or were obtaining psychoanalytic training had shrunk from 89 to 66. In addition, a smaller proportion than in the first years came into the program with psychoanalytic training behind them.

During this period, the criteria for supplementing a developmental award with funds to support psychoanalytic training remained essentially unchanged. However, the issue was so important, the cost so great, and a number of doubts so persistent that much time was devoted to examining many aspects of psychoanalysis in psychiatry in general and in the Research Development Program in particular.

Thus participants at the Career Investigator Conference held in 1965 tried to appraise the role of psychoanalysis. (The details of that appraisal cannot be discussed here, but the gross outline can communicate something of the flavor of the deliberations.)

Participants listed valuable contributions of psychoanalysis and psychoanalysts. First, psychoanalysis had offered a means of understanding unconscious processes, the psychology of self-deception, and the widespread discrepancy between public standards and private wishes. Second, it had promoted a serious interest in the psychology of motivation and emotion. Third, psychoanalysis had revealed the great significance of earlier experience for the character of later, adult behavior. Fourth, it had promoted the detailed longitudinal study of the individual, including those aspects usually under social taboo, thus serving as a foundation for modern developmental psychology. Fifth, it had pointed to the signal function of anxiety and the defense mechanisms against it. Sixth, it had provided insights into the relations between loss, grief, and depression that would not have been available without it.

Participants at the conference also discussed the limitations of psychoanalysis. Psychoanalysis was said to have acquired an institutional, static quality that was conservative and dogmatic, to lack research vitality, and to have quasi-religious aspects. Over the years it had grown to encompass a narrow spectrum of private practice and, in the process, had become isolated from medicine and science. This condition was reflected in a different set of values between psychoanalysis, on the one hand, and either science or medicine, on the other. Accumulated clinical evidence in the years since the original development of psychoanalysis began to provoke questions concerning many of the theoretical hypotheses of psychoanalysis. The usefulness of this approach was limited by the time, expense, and energy it required of the therapist as well as of his eventual patients. Finally, psychoanalysis avoided dealing with the seriously ill.

Given this general balance of assets and liabilities, the group tried to assess how important psychoanalysis was as an element of research training for a mental health research career. On the positive side was the orientation to important issues, especially to the detailed study of the individual. On the negative side were the time and energy involved, the intellectual isolation, and the growing concern that, while psychoanalysis might aid in clinical practice, it might in some respects be antithetical to a research career. At this point the group decided that they needed information beyond their own experiences—specifically, a study of the issues involved in the role of psychoanalysis in research training.

*The 1966 Study of Psychoanalytic Training for Research.*   In December 1965, the Selection Committee approved initiating a relatively informal study of psychoanalytic training as preparation for research on problems relevant to clinical psychiatry. Twenty-nine research scientists were asked to complete a questionnaire; all of these scientists had psychoanalytic experience and had sustained an active program of research for periods of 8 to over 20 years. Psychiatrists in the midst of psychoanalytic training, personal analysis, or seminars were not included. The group was told that the Selection Committee members were considering a number of issues: whether the full training program required for psychoanalytic practice is appropriate to the development of a research scientist; whether the time and energy required for traditional psychoanalytic training creates unnecessary stress during a period of special importance in the development of a research career; and whether the various peripheral benefits of psychoanalytic training, when research involves neither psychoanalytic hypotheses nor psychoanalytic methods, are sufficient to justify the large investment required.

The letter asking for personal information and advice contained the following assurance and statement of purpose:

> In 1966, as in 1954 at the beginning of the program, the Reviewing Committee [also known as the Selection Committee] wishes to encourage the best possible candidates to undertake careers of research on problems relevant to clinical psychiatry, and there is no inclination to recommend any withdrawal or restriction of support for relevant training of recognized value. With respect to psychoanalytic training, the Committee believes that it is time, in other words that sufficient experience has been accumulated, to make some improved evaluation of how it functions in the research career program.

The investigators were invited to comment freely on their own psychoanalytic training and to generalize about its value. They were encouraged, but not requested, to comment an a variety of issues: contribution of their training to their professional development, influence of the investigator's psychoanalytic training on experimental work, and how the research scientist viewed conventional methods of psychoanalytic training. Nine leading psychiatric educators and research scientists with psychoanalytic experience who were familiar with the NIMH Research Career Program were also asked to contribute their views. Twenty-four of the group of 29 investigators responded, as did seven of the nine educators.

Of the 24 investigators who responded, 17 were psychiatrists, six were psychologists, and one was an internist with considerable experience in a psychiatric setting. The extent of psychoanalytic experience among the members of the group varied considerably. Seven had not gone beyond personal analysis to other formal aspects of psychoanalytic training. Eight had engaged in considerable psychoanalytic study beyond personal analysis, with more or less participation in psychoanalytic seminars, in control cases, or in both. Nine had completed psychoanalytic training as directed by the psychoanalytic institutes. In their research, 15 of the 24 worked on clinical problems with human subjects, and nine did laboratory work with non-human subjects. All but two of the nine said they planned to move into the study of clinical problems requiring human subjects.

Most of the opinions from this research group were summarized in relation to general professional development (meaning both personal effectiveness and professional knowledge and skill), the influence of psychoanalytic experience on research work, and the effectiveness of conventional methods in psychoanalytic training.

*The Contribution of Psychoanalysis to Personal Development and Professional Education.* Of the 24 investigators, 22 commented on their psychoanalytic training in relation to personal well-being or effectiveness, professional education, or professional competence. Fifteen wrote specifically about the role of psychoanalytic training, particularly personal analysis, in enabling them to overcome personal problems. With one exception, they were strongly positive that psychoanalysis had contributed significantly to personal well-being and effectiveness. Sixteen of the 24 investigators commented positively on the value of psychoanalysis in their professional education. For eight of the group, psychoanalytic study was considered essential—the central if not the main part of their psychiatric education. Others spoke of the value of psychoanalysis in clinical work and in communication with colleagues. Two of the investigators had only very faint praise for psychoanalytic training, one saying that it *might* help with personal problems and another that it *might* improve clinical skill. There was one opinion of a quite different character—namely, that the discernable benefit of psychoanalytic training was socioeconomic.

*The Value of Psychoanalysis in Psychiatric Research.* All except one of the Career Investigators discussed psychoanalytic training in relation to their own experimental work. In their evaluation of psychoanalysis as preparation for research, some were enthusiastic and unqualified in their praise; some recognized a value, but not an essential value, to research; and some felt either that there was no direct contribution of psychoanalysis to research or that psychoanalytic training was of dubious value if not destructive to the work of a research scientist. The majority of the group were either firmly positive that psychoanalytic training has a high value in research or disinterestedly of the opinion that it may have some value.

For at least seven of the group, their research was a natural outgrowth of their psychoanalytic scholarship. Psychoanalysis was their main scientific frame of reference; they believed that the research that they had already done and wished to do in the future would have been inconceivably or hopelessly handicapped if they had not had psychoanalytic knowledge and skills. The following statement was characteristic of this group of seven: "Psychoanalysis is indispensable for the study of clinical phenomena, research in personality, and research on human behavior." One of the seven specified that such training would not be worthwhile for a scientist whose research would not require psychoanalytic theory and methodology. Two of this group pointed out that the advancement of psychoanalytic theory must depend on the work of research scientists; they expressed their hope that psychiatrists developing research careers would continue to complete psychoanalytic training and use it in their research. Seven other investigators wrote positively about psychoanalytic training, but without the enthusiasm of the first group of seven. Members of the second group believed either that psychoanalytic training was invaluable in clinical research, that it was theoretically valuable in any study of development, that it was useful for research in personality, or that it had some value in the development of clinical skills for use in clinical research.

Another group of four valued psychoanalytic training but at the same time expressed reservations. One respondent said that psychoanalytic training was valuable in studies of human behavior, but he also thought that his indecision in contemplating new projects and the continuation of his career as a research scientist had been produced by his psychoanalytic training. Two of the investigators who recognized that the training may be worthwhile either for research based on psychoanalytic hypotheses or in clinical experiments nonetheless considered it likely to cause bias or loss of scientific motivation. One of the more senior investigators who discussed the value of psychoanalytic training in developmental research also cautioned that it may narrow an investigator's interest.

Two of the scientists stated simply that they had been able to see no value in a psychoanalytic background for research, although one of these two hoped to use his psychoanalytic training in his future research.

Three investigators had definitely negative opinions. One believed that the results of psychoanalytic training are unpredictable: for some the result may be supportive in a research career, but others may be irresistibly attracted away from research. One investigator stated his belief that on the whole, psychoanalytic training undermines a psychiatrist's interest in research; and one of the senior investigators believed that, in general, it has a deterrent effect on experimental work.

The 23 opinions may be summarized as seven strongly favoring psychoanalytic training for research; seven favoring psychoanalytic training for research in specified areas; four ambivalent in recognition of definite positive and negative effects; two noncommital beyond saying that psychoanalysis had not been helpful in the investigator's own research; and three mainly or definitely negative.

*Opinions on Conventional Psychoanalytic Training.*    Opinions on the nature of psychoanalytic training as the investigators had experienced or perceived it were more sharply divided than comments on the value of psychoanalysis. Eighteen of the 24 investigators mentioned the pattern of psychoanalytic training represented by the psychoanalytic institutes. Eight of the group approved of this pattern, whereas 10 believed it to be defective at least for research scientists' training. Of the approving group, seven considered that all three parts of institute psychoanalytic training—training analysis, seminars, and supervised practice—were essential, and that they had unquestionably benefited from the whole course of the experience. There were few qualifications to these comments. One said that without strong personal motivation, psychoanalytic training would be wasteful. One recognized that the psychoanalytic curriculum may have grown too much by accretion and that careful study might refine it. A third recognized that some modification might be advisable for the research scientist. Ten of the investigators believed that orthodox methods of psychoanalytic training were inadequate. The most frequently expressed opinion is that the training was excessive, much of it inappropriate with respect to the maturity and ability of the candidates, or unsuitable, particularly for a research scientist. Three investigators simply commented that both seminars and control cases should be greatly reduced, and one recommended subsuming all psychoanalytic training under the three-year psychiatric residency program. Several commented that individual study was superior to the seminar method, with its prescribed reading, lectures or group discussions, and weekly meetings. Others commented on lack of competence among psychoanalytic teachers; one had found them unscholarly and not scientifically objective. A few said that the cost in time and energy of full psychoanalytic training was disproportionate to its value. Two of the investigators believed that no formal training was helpful beyond the personal analysis. One was opposed to the major content of the training as injurious to the intellectual development of a research scientist.

*Additional Comments from Teachers of Psychiatry and Psychoanalysis.*    Of the nine psychiatric educators who were invited to comment on the value of psychoanalytic training, seven responded; two sent copies of papers they had written on the subject. All expressed their approval of an inquiry into the opinions of research scientists. One, while recognizing the value of the knowledge that would be obtained from such a group, urged the Selection Committee to interpret the results as no more than tentative. He believed that it was too early to see clear results of psychoanalytic backgrounds in the work of psychiatric investigators.

Four of the consultants believed that research conditioned and motivated by psychoanalytic training would materially advance psychiatric knowledge and that it should be whole-heartedly supported. To one of the group, psychoanalytic thinking is an essential dimension in studies of human behavior, and the full training is required for the proper balance of knowledge and skill in such research. In the view of this educator, improvements in training must be worked out with great caution by teachers in the psychoanalytic institutes.

Another consultant, equally convinced that psychoanalytic knowledge and skills were essential in psychiatric research, stressed the importance of motivation by personal need in personal analysis; he asserted that clinical practice under supervision is second in importance only to the personal analysis, because the latter brings verbal concepts into reality. He believed, however, that the didactic programs of the institutes are based on a childish system which he described as rigid, regressive, and far too time-consuming.

One of the consultants submitted a paper based on a questionnaire sent in 1961 to about 75 behavioral scientists with psychoanalytic experience. Of the 49 who completed the questionnaire, 82 percent believed that the experience of personal analysis had benefited them personally and professionally. For the 28 behavioral scientists who had completed their didactic training, their evaluations of lecture courses and seminars were tabulated. Ratings of 92 courses were distributed as follows: 41 high, 32 medium, and 19 low. This consultant also included a paper he had written on possibilities of improving the teaching of psychoanalysis, reasoning that if it were brought into the university milieu, it would be subject to critical evaluation and analysis together with other psychological systems.

One consultant favored personal analysis as an adjunct to clinical training and to psychoanalytic theory because of its value to the psychodynamic understanding of patients, but he believed that beyond personal analysis, formal training is a waste of time. He also thought that formal psychoanalytic training is hazardous because it conveys prejudice against research.

Another consultant doubted whether the time and energy psychoanalytic training required were justified. In his view, all aspects of psychoanalytic training were excessive. The final consultant felt that much

research is needed to clarify and define the scope of psychoanalysis in relation to other approaches to clinical practice. Psychoanalysis for him was only
one approach, the results of which are mainly untested.

   *1967–1973.*   The doubts and limitations expressed in 1966 appear to have proved prophetic. While the Selection Committee continued
to be permissive in approving funds for psychoanalytic training as a part of
research training (the first rejection of such a supplemental request in the
history of the Committee occurred in 1972), the proportion of prospective
candidates requesting such funds continued to drop. As may be seen in
Table 2, the decline has been persistent and substantial. For comparison
with the figures in Table 2, recall that for the period 1954–1960, the percentage with psychoanalytic training was 89 percent, while for the period
1961–1966 it had been 66 percent.

*Table 2.*   Numbers and Percentages of Type I Awardees
Receiving Support for Psychoanalytic Training since
July, 1966

|  | Number of Type I Awards | Number in Psychoanalytic Training | Percentage |
|---|---|---|---|
| 1967 | 37 | 18 | 50 |
| 1968 | 35 | 12 | 35 |
| 1969 | 35 | 9 | 26 |
| 1970 | 30 | 6 | 20 |
| 1971 | 30 | 6 | 20 |
| 1972 | 31 | 7 | 23 |
| 1973 | 25 | 4 | 16 |

   Among the 15 Level I awardees discussed earlier, seven took
psychoanalytic training as a part of their psychiatric and research training
and described their experiences and the role and value of their psychoanalytic training. The following excerpts give some impression of the range
of values these seven individuals attribute to their training:

   Now I am in the third year of classes at the ——— Psychoanalytic Institute and am seeing two cases of supervised psychoanalysis.
Psychoanalytic training provides a view of behavior that otherwise
would simply not be available. I feel this view is indispensable. The
training is providing me with a sophistication about analytic theory
and also with improved skills, but the unique exposure to complex
behavior is particularly important.

   I feel that psychoanalysis has been a central part of my development. . . . I feel it has enormously deepened and broadened my
clinical perspectives and ultimately will lead to a greater relevance

of my research data to clinical problems of development and disease
states. . . . Psychoanalytic training provided additional invaluable
experience. My didactic analysis not only increased my self-knowl-
edge in terms of my early development and in other areas but also
freed up energy. Supervision of control cases and psychoanalytic
seminars has provided an understanding of the psychoanalytic techniques as a research and clinical tool. In addition, participating in
seminars at the ———— Psychoanalytic Institute has provided an
understanding of consistencies and inconsistencies of psychoanalytic
theory and has led to some developing abilities to evaluate data from
the psychoanalytic clinical setting.

Psychoanalysis was the theory at the core of my psychiatric training, and it played a significant role as devil's advocate in the conflict
between "hard" and "soft" science. I was never tempted by the
possibility of a full-time psychoanalytic practice. Although I was
considered a good analyst by others, I have never fully trusted my
own skills or the results or formulations of the practice of psychoanalysis. I became seriously disillusioned, not with the theory itself
but with its practitioners. At the same time I have become convinced that psychoanalytic theory is not a fruitful basis for the study
of human development except in very limited areas. Most research
efforts using psychoanalytic techniques seem to me rank failures,
and the best use I could make of my psychoanalytic training has
been very personal.

The need to be quite devoted to [psychoanalytic] training over a
long period of time made it impossible [for me] to leave the area for
a year or two. I, therefore, could not go to the ———— program for
training in research and psychiatry for a year or to another university
center away from the area without [appreciably disrupting my] psychoanalytic training. Since my research is on conscious experience
of thought, imagery, and emotion, psychoanalytic training seemed
to be of great relevance to me and became a more important commitment. Because of this difficulty, my own training in research
methodology became a relatively autonomous project. I learned
more by trial and error than by planned learning. For me, . . .
psychoanalytic training has been worthwhile because it has given
me confidence in my ability to work clinically with conscious experience. It has also provided me with a theoretical context for my
research interests. While I thus estimate it to be valuable to me in
my training, it did take enormous chunks of time since there was a
lot of reading for seminars, the seminars themselves, the training
analysis, transportation to and from the training analysis, supervision, and [the] clinical experience of doing psychoanalysis. This
expenditure of time in psychoanalytic training reduces somewhat
the energy and time available for struggling with research issues.
It slows down research development. While research development
is slower, it may reach a greater level of sophistication with this
training, however. My personal evaluation is that I am at the end

of eight years of a Research Development Award, just arriving at a position to do clearly focused, independent, and scientifically worthwhile research. I think that my investigations so far have been valuable, but there have also been many blind alleys. These blind alleys are a part of research, but the number of them entered, I think, can be reduced by anticipatory learning.

I was convinced that the psychoanalytic method was the only true way to comprehend the meaning of dream content. I am sure that is why my application requested a supplement for psychoanalysis and avoided other training possibilities.

Speaking frankly, I see now that psychoanalytic training was "rationalized" as research training to some degree. The fact was that I needed financial assistance for psychoanalysis in view of the income restrictions of the ... Award. I still saw myself, at the time, becoming a psychoanalyst, and at the very least wanted to have excellent institute training in psychoanalysis. . . .

The psychoanalytic supplement allowed me to straddle the fence [between research and a career as a psychoanalyst]. . . .

What has changed, certainly, is the belief in or reliance on psychoanalytic tools.

Of course, psychiatric skills always help me to deal with subjects and patients in my research and, in a few studies, have helped me to evaluate the data. It is so much a part of me, perhaps I am in danger of underestimating how much I use it. But even in the area of dream content my psychiatric, not psychoanalytic, training has been called on. . . . Though these relationships were clearly of interest to Freud and may eventually be helpful to psychoanalysts toward understanding the links between waking life and dream life, the connections will be indirect in terms of their interest. For we are looking for formal and quantifiable derivatives of perception in the manifest content of dreams, not attempting in any respect to look at latent meaning.

I also underwent some years of psychoanalytic training. which I did not find to be as useful as I had hoped but nevertheless an asset.

The last respondent wrote that psychoanalytic training had taken him precisely in the wrong directions; he detailed the great difficulty he had in overcoming the deleterious effects of his training in psychoanalytic theory and principles. Unlearning for him was a much harder process than learning. He concluded:

Undoing what my psychiatric training had done was the hardest thing for me. There must be some way not to do it to the young professional in the first place.

Perhaps the observation of a prominent chairman of a major department of psychiatry who has served on the program's Review Committee is not too harsh when he says:

> My own impression is that the psychoanalytic training contributed nothing toward the psychiatrist's development as a research worker and in most cases had a deleterious effect ranging from mild to severe.

The preceding comments were stimulated by what might be termed a social experiment. When the Research Development Program was initiated in the mid-1950s (then called the Career Investigator Grant program), psychoanalysis had a pre-eminent place in American psychiatry. Its value for the research scientist remained to be tested, however. Arguments could have been advanced on either side, but an objective assessment of its efficacy was impossible at that time. By providing generous support, the Research Development Program allowed a full exploration of the potential for research of psychoanalysis and psychoanalytic training. As the previously quoted chairman expressed it:

> These forms of training were evaluated in the crucible of experience and found wanting; [they were] simply abandoned for lack of apparent value for research in psychiatry. Without such generous support, it seems to me quite likely that we would still be listening to battles between pro- and anti-psychoanalysis adversaries, and we would still be wondering what could have happened had this promising field received the support that some felt was its due.

Thus, if the evidence now indicates that the effects of psychoanalytic training are frequently negative for a research career, the knowledge gained from the experiment is nonetheless useful for future investigators and their advisors. It might also lead psychoanalytic institutions to reexamine their practices and assumptions in dealing with research-oriented young investigators.

# Toward the Future of Psychiatric Science

## 5

The Research Development Program was initiated in response to one of the most widespread and acknowledged social needs: to decrease the enormous social and financial cost of mental illness in our society. It has sought to establish a research base for the mental health professions, primarily psychiatry, because this branch of medicine was almost alone in its lack of significant scientific breakthroughs that had materially improved the health of mankind.

The Research Development Program was born, like some federal programs, because perceptive, forward-looking individuals saw a need and devised a feasible, intelligent way of responding to it with available financial and human resources. (See Chapter 6, History of the Research Development Program.) The program reflects the collective wisdom of federal administrators, academic scientists, and practitioners who had long worked and exchanged views together and had their fingers on the pulse of academic psychiatry and related scientific disciplines. It is the product of wise intuition guided by a good feedback system from awardees, institutions, departmental chairmen, and consultants. How much progress has been made toward reaching its goals? And, in light of its long history, how may further progress be stimulated? These two questions will be discussed next.

## The Impact of the Research Development Program

The experience of the Research Development Program generally has been profoundly satisfying for its federal sponsors, for the scientists it has supported, and for the psychiatric service institutions it has affected. In the period 1954–1972, the federal government has supported 324 individuals in mental health research through the Research Development Program. Of these, 179 worked in departments of psychiatry and other psychiatric institutions. During the same time, psychiatry has taken a significant step toward becoming a science as well as an art. Many psychiatrists and other behavioral scientists now view a career in full-time psychiatric research as a legitimate alternative to clinical and academic pursuits. Still others see psychiatric research as a vital component of their professional life style, albeit less than a full-time pursuit. There are now esteemed, productive psychiatric scientists working and teaching in major medical schools throughout the country. In 1967, in approximately half of the medical schools in the United States, one or more research psychiatrists held faculty positions. The number has undoubtedly grown since then.

> Among all American institutions and agencies there are well over 150 psychiatrists experienced in research who maintain their identity as research psychiatrists in a variety of influential positions. They are appointed to a full range of academic positions. They serve as chiefs of laboratories and as directors of programs in hospitals and institutes. Some of these investigators are chairmen of university departments or the directors of large state or federal institutions [Group for the Advancement of Psychiatry, 1967].

Dr. Boothe estimated that in 1972 there were about 250 full-time psychiatric research scientists in the United States, of whom about 200 were supported by the Research Development Program.

A high proportion of scientists who have received Research Development Program support have become leading figures in their fields and have made major contributions to psychiatric science. For example, within NIMH, an assessment was made in 1973 of the extent to which the Institute's support has furthered the biological sciences relevant to understanding mental health and illness. Twenty-five active leaders in the field were asked to reflect on progress over the past 25 years in their special areas of interest, to note landmark studies, and to identify outstanding individuals. Recipients of NIMH Research Development Awards figured prominently among the notable scientists who were mentioned. Of the approximately 300 former and current Research Development Program awardees, about one-third had been working in biological science areas relevant to mental health. Of these, a majority were found to have made significant contributions to their field.

The 1973 awardee list was then studied to assess current contributions. As one reviewer put it, "Looking over the list, name after name would be considered not only to have contributed significantly, but to be a prime mover of research, leading the way." He then cited specific individual contributions. For example, one basic scientist who has received some 10 years of support from the program has done "magnificent research on brain chemistry" that has resulted in a "breakthrough" demonstrating an anatomical basis for shifts in concentrations of biogenic amines in the brain. Such information helps to establish a firm scientific foundation for psychopharmacology and may eventually aid in understanding and correcting chemical abnormalities underlying mental illness. Another scientist has for many years explored the anatomical connectivities of the brain, particularly the limbic system; he has developed both techniques and concepts that serve as the basis for many current studies of memory and emotional behavior. His work, again, provides a cornerstone for innumerable others who are attempting to understand the physical foundations of the psyche.

The intrinsic abilities of grantees, their education, the support of their departments and colleagues, as well as the private, state, and federal funds that have also paid for their research have all contributed to the grantees' success and stature. In addition, the fellowship programs and extramural research grant programs of NIMH have supported many of these scientists before, during, and after their contact with the Research Development Program. Yet, as many of the awardees have acknowledged, only through long-term, full-salary support from the Research Development Program could they have made the major commitment to research needed for scientific excellence.

The presence of these outstanding scientists in medical and graduate departments throughout the country has meant that their work has had double value. Their investigations, life styles, and scientific approaches have inspired their fellow scientists and have served as a model for younger scientists, many of whom will choose research careers themselves or will incorporate in their clinical practice the tough-minded curiosity of their scientist teachers.

*Departmental Impact.* In medical schools and hospitals throughout the country there are now several departments of psychiatry that are centers of research excellence. For most, their growth in research strength has been relatively recent, within the past 10 or 20 years. It reflects the tendency of psychiatry to become more of an academic discipline like all other branches of medicine (in which research, like teaching and clinical service, is an essential departmental component); this growth also reflects the influence of the Research Development Program.

By supporting more than one and often several investigators in research-receptive psychiatry departments, the Research Development Program has provided such departments with the nucleus of a research staff. The grantees in these institutions, through the merit of their work and the status in part conferred by the program's support, have in turn attracted a host of other research scientists with various forms of support. Not only have many psychiatric departments grown in the amount and quality of research but the character of their teaching and clinical activities has also been affected by their strengthened research activities. Students from a host of disciplines—both practice- and research-oriented—are taught by the research faculty and see them as models. In addition, professional colleagues are affected by their interchanges, both formal and informal, with the research staff.

The following comments by chairmen of several departments of psychiatry that have developed a strong research base (with the help of the Research Development Program) indicate the synergistic effects of having numerous scientists of different disciplines working in the same environment dedicated to the common goal of understanding and preventing the causes of mental illness and providing more effective treatment for the mentally ill.

The overall departmental impact of the Research Development Program is summarized by one department chairman as follows:

> There is no question that the program has had an impact on departments and has provided monies for the support of people who are interested in doing psychiatric research. It has had an effect on departments in terms of teaching and training in that medical students, residents, and fellows have been put in contact with those who are scientifically inclined and think in terms of doing experiments on important clinical and scientific problems. It has also allowed the establishment of strong research departments in about six to ten departments of psychiatry throughout the country. Without the lever of the program, I think it would have been impossible to do this, especially as there is a strong clinical tradition in departments of psychiatry and no great [incentive for] doing research in the field. Because of the prestige of the program and the provision of monies to set it up, it has been possible to attract people in departments of psychiatry who are primarily interested in doing research in the field. It has also allowed them to become trained in areas relevant to psychiatry and to bring various techniques to bear on the enormous clinical problems that exist in the field. It has been possible by these means, then, to develop departments of psychiatry that are very much more akin to other clinical departments in the medical school in that many young people, following their clinical training, do take fellowship training very often under the guidance and supervision of persons who are supported by the Research Development Program.

In describing the impact of the program on their particular departments, several department chairmen have acknowledged the substantial contribution of the program to their growth. For example, as one noted:

> Since the program began, there have been 11 recipients of an award from NIMH, and two recipients of an award from NIH. Without these 13 awards, the department would not be able to be as productive in active research and to become known as a research department of psychiatry. The areas covered by persons who have received these awards include clinical psychiatry, sociology, epidemiology, neuropsychiatry, electronmicroscopy, and neuropsychology. . . . These awards have also permitted us to have a very diverse and yet intensive program in a number of different areas. Of the 11 persons who received NIMH awards, nine of them were trained psychiatrists, one was a psychologist, and one a sociologist. . . .
> Without these awards the department would not have been able to grow or produce, for example, the 213 research papers published in the past two years and the slightly fewer than 200 published in the two years prior to that. I believe that having [this many awardees] . . . has given this department a strong and long-lasting impetus toward productive investigative work. . . . My belief is that the Research Development Program is probably the single most successful program that has been initiated by the NIH or NIMH. . . .

Another chairman has expressed similar comments concerning his institution:

> . . . Without the Research Development Program, there would have been far less basic and clinical research at our institution in recent years. The level of financial support from the University and the state, in combination with the administrative, teaching, and service demands, [has] precluded the high level of research activities made possible by the Research Development Program. But even more important has been the inestimable value to our institution of the spin-off, in terms of teaching and clinical practice, that derives from having a significant core of full-time investigators with the freedom to explore.

Several chairmen, in discussing the program's impact, have mentioned its specific effects on other faculty members, on students, and on the quality of clinical service in their departments. Faculty impact was described by one chairman as follows:

> There has been a mutual interplay between the persons who have received awards and those members of the department who have not received awards so that there is no member of the department

who currently spends less than one-third of his time in research, and a good many spend up to 75 percent of their time in research even though they do not have an award.

Another chairman explained that both faculty members and students have benefited:

> Individuals either currently supported by or having had past support from the program have had a pronounced effect on research productivity in psychiatry at our institution. This is particularly true in the area of newer, more innovative mental health research activities, both biological and sociopsychological. The names of investigators who have been or who are currently supported by awards appear in published research findings with remarkable frequency. Their co-authors reflect the spread of their influence. All are involved in truly interdisciplinary basic and clinically relevant research that has involved a wide range of fellow faculty, students, and other trainees. All have had psychiatric residents, medical students, psychology fellows, nursing and social work students, and other health professionals either working or consulting with them. Without question, each has provided an excellent model for a wide range of students in many disciplines.

Grantees' educational impact has been described by another chairman:

> The influence of the Research Development Program on research has also influenced the teaching programs of our institution. The people in the research areas have become so numerous and so influential in the department and their special knowledge so valuable that they have become important faculty members for students and residents in the development of the teaching program. This holds true not only for the research-oriented trainee but also for the trainee in general psychiatry.

One chairman said that awardees' studies affected the quality of clinical care when the studies evolved to a stage at which their influence spread from the laboratory to the clinic and back to the laboratory. For instance:

> 1. Dr. ———, who was initially involved in animal neurophysiology research, has developed new electrophysiological techniques useful in the diagnosis of psychomotor epilepsy and in the treatment of anxiety. This has evolved from close collaboration with the outpatient staffs of the Departments of Neurosurgery and Psychiatry. The freedom to change research directions led to this successful marriage of basic science and clinical investigators.

2. Dr. ———— has been able to apply psychophysiological techniques and concepts useful in the diagnosis of schizophrenia to studies of altered states of consciousness induced by a variety of abused drugs, thereby leading to a more general understanding of both naturally occurring and drug-induced psychotic states.

3. Dr. ————'s basic studies of nonverbal behavior have led to a number of clinically relevant diagnostic and training techniques related to facial expression and other nonverbal communication patterns. This investigator has devised a remarkable technique and instrumentation for frame-by-frame analysis of videotape.

This chairman credited many of these clinically relevant advances to the freedom and flexibility afforded by the program's support:

> The freedom for the investigator provided by the program has been a great advantage to the Department of Psychiatry. It has allowed the investigators to shift the emphasis of their activities to meet rapidly changing social and scientific demands. This freedom has allowed them the opportunity to explore new, innovative approaches to the solution of mental health problems.

Another chairman, whose department research group has been directed by one of the first Career Investigators, notes that:

> ... under [that grantee's] direction, it was possible to build up a serious, broad-spectrum research group [that] covered a range of investigative interests from largely biological and neurophysiological research to psychological and social research.... That group of research workers became nationally prominent and served as an enormous stimulus to scholarship, increased breadth of vision, and ultimately improved patient care in our Division of Psychiatry.... The backbone of this group was a group of investigators supported by the Research Development Program. Without that program, the advances and their consequent impact on psychiatry, both here and at wider, national levels, would not have been possible.

This chairman cited the work of a number of individual grantees and their influence on the department's growth and quality. For example:

> Dr. ———— has continued to be a pioneer in psychosomatic and psychoanalytic investigation. He has been chairman of research committees in psychoanalytic societies and has had a continuous impact in bringing scientific methods to bear on clinical psychiatric material.
>
> Early in the course of developing a research program at our university, we were able to recruit Dr. ————. It would not have been possible to secure his services without the Research Development Program. He has been continuously supported by it and has been

an outstanding investigator, contributing basic knowledge to our understanding of arousal mechanisms in his work with both humans and monkeys. He has investigated perinatal and neonatal injuries and their possible role in schizophrenia. He has excited a generation of medical students and stimulated a number of residents to undertake research projects with him. At the same time he has been nationally prominent in a number of societies and in the Review Committees of the NIMH. His impact has been powerful both within and outside our medical school. . . .

Dr. ———— is another example of an outstanding, original, creative individual who has had a national and international impact, as well as being a thoughtful teacher to small groups of medical students and residents and a sponsor for a number of research trainees. [His] career would have been utterly impossible without the Research Development Program award. His approach is unusual, involving naturalistic models rather than the conventional experimental ones. In addition, he is a thoughtful and scholarly individual who needed time to find his own identity as a researcher. If he had had to rely on conventional grant support, his steady development toward research excellence would have been sacrificed.

In summing up the program's impact on his department, this chairman reiterated the philosophy that has kindled and sustained the entire Research Development Program:

It is clear that the commitment implied by the award [means] not only . . . long-range stability but an equal commitment on the part of the recipient. He is pledged to a research career. The stimulus of competitive renewal remains with him, but he is not bound by discrete projects and forced to shift according to the fate of particular experiments or the changes in climate of granting agencies. If one seriously believes, as we do, that advance in health care cannot take place without new discoveries, one must be convinced that the investment in a manpower base from which such discoveries may come is a solid [one]. No one . . . recipient can produce guaranteed results. Discovery is always a matter, to a certain extent, of good fortune and rare combinations of talent. Nevertheless, I suggest that the experience at our institution shows how a climate centering around a number of outstanding investigators can have an overall profoundly beneficial effect on the course of a particular . . . sector of psychiatry.

The net impact of progress in many departments throughout the country has been a change in the overall research climate in psychiatry. There have, of course, been many causes for this change, but the Research Development Program has unquestionably been a significant force. As one department chairman put it:

The first major impact that the program has had has been on the field. In the course of the last 15 years there has certainly been a clear-cut impact of the program on research activities in psychiatry. It was fortunate, perhaps, that the program came at a time when there was much astir in the fields of neurochemistry and neuropharmacology, which in turn was generated by the use of the various pharmacological agents in the treatment of the major psychoses. It is now apparent that there is a clearly identifiable nucleus of about 100 to 150 people in the field who are doing respectable work, whereas before, the field was not exactly known for the rigor of its scientific work. Much of the credit for the establishment of a research base in the field of psychiatry belongs to the program and to the "halo effect" of the people in the program on others in the field.

## Preconditions for Progress

How can the future development of psychiatric science and new generations of mental health researchers be further encouraged? The experience of the Research Development Program has shown that certain conditions seem to favor productive careers in psychiatric research. These include: (1) a reward system that provides sufficient status, security, and salary to promising, productive scientists; (2) a setting that stimulates creative research and teaching and fosters cross-disciplinary communication as well as an interchange between researcher and clinician; and (3) an educational system that provides adequate opportunities for students to gain extensive first-hand research experience as well as exposure to both clinical and scientific skills and attitudes necessary for psychiatric research.

1. *The Reward System.* Scientific research is a slow, tedious, painstaking occupation that leads to many more blind alleys than great discoveries. For those who enjoy the quest, as research scientists must, the search and the hope of discovery are the primary rewards. Yet even scientists whose primary motivation is intellectual are moved at critical decision points in their career by such mundane considerations as salaries, status, and security. If mental health research is to attract and keep scientists of superior training and talent, such rewards should be available and compare favorably with those in competing areas of endeavor.

For medically trained scientists, a research salary will inevitably compare poorly with income from private practice. In addition, in academic life, whatever the discipline, the reward system is too often all or nothing: tenured professors have status, security, and relatively high salaries; non-tenured faculty, especially those doing research, must scratch for a living as best they can. Judging by the comments of Research Development Program grantees, the program has improved their situation somewhat, providing at least more security than is usually available to a research scientist, a respectable salary, and a degree of status.

Yet for those in psychiatric settings, especially behavioral scientists, the situation is particularly difficult. Academic prestige in psychiatry is still based largely on clinical rather than scientific skills, and rewards are distributed accordingly. Since psychiatry departments rarely give full-time research scientists top priority in their staffing decisions, in times of tight money, like the present, department support vanishes. Thus, the research scientist—be he psychiatrist, behavioral scientist, neuroscientist, or psycho-pharmacologist—is a welcome member of many psychiatry departments only so long as he pays his own way. In the future, it is possible that as research begins to have more visible clinical applications, the situation may change; priorities may be altered somewhat, but this is likely to be a slow process.

Psychiatry does not have a long research tradition, and research is not yet built into the expectations-and-reward system as it is, say, in departments of psychology. Medical school deans and psychiatry department chairmen will thus continue to play a pivotal role in encouraging research in psychiatry. If their commitment to research can be translated into developing ways to provide status, adequate salary, and security for researchers, both medical and nonmedical, then psychiatric research can continue to flourish.

2. *The Setting.* Mental health research is currently being carried out in a variety of settings, including medical school basic science departments, mental hospitals, graduate departments of psychology and biological sciences, and university-affiliated and independent research institutions. This rich diversity should be maintained although the program's experience has underscored the importance of conducting mental health research in a clinically oriented setting. If there is physical proximity to and interaction with clinical workers, mutually beneficial collaboration is stimulated, research information and attitudes may be more readily disseminated to clinicians and their students, and researchers can keep abreast of pressing clinical needs and problems bearing on practice.

3. *The Scientist: Character and Training.* The most essential requirement for the future of any research is a growing corps of superior young scientists. Psychiatric research demands not only the usual prerequisites for scientific research—intelligence, determination, patience—but also a sensitivity to the rich nuances and complex repertoire of human

behavior in sickness and health; especially in clinical research, the scientist's rigor and objectivity must be reconciled with the clinician's sympathetic and humane perspective.

The essential characteristics needed for psychiatric research are often seen as a research orientation. This can and should be identified and stimulated early in a student's education, whatever his discipline, so he has every opportunity to develop to his full ability. Although one can become a superior mental health research scientist whatever his background or formal discipline—M.D., Ph.D., psychiatrist, psychologist, or biochemist—if he has the right research instincts and experience, formal education and training can unquestionably help or hinder his growth. Unfortunately, the present structure of the professional educational system tends to encourage those who are research oriented to become Ph.D. scientists, not M.D.s. Graduate schools then further exaggerate the differences between the physician's pragmatic, human-healing involvement and the scientist's skeptical detachment. Professional custom and legal requirements further expand the gap between scientist and practitioner, since only medically trained personnel are allowed access to the primary focus of mental health research: the human patient.

One essential lesson from the Research Development Program has been that research is learned largely by doing, over and over, under the guidance of teachers who themselves are research scientists. The process is best started early. Thus, research-oriented undergraduates and graduate students, as well as medical students, should be given adequate opportunities to do research themselves. The Psychiatry Panel of the Behavioral and Social Sciences Survey reported their suggestions on starting students in actual research (Hamburg, 1970). Research training could take the form of psychiatrically relevant research programs introduced in undergraduate and social science graduate departments as well as basic science or behavioral science research electives during medical school. Research experience can also be encouraged at higher levels of professional education. For example, a research fellowship could be offered to medical trainees between internship and residency. Similarly, elective time for psychiatric residents could be expanded for research training. After residency or doctoral training, research fellowships can help the developing research scientist explore promising leads and test his career choice. At the highest level of professional postgraduate training, programs such as the Research Development Program can provide support for the full development of a research career.

If the educational system retains its two paths (M.D. and Ph.D.) to research careers, the two paths must be encouraged to converge much more than they do now, both in content and in orientation. One approach is to train a new breed of scientific psychiatrists. If research-oriented college graduates sense that a respected, rewarding career can be found in psychiatric research, and if they are made more welcome in medical schools and psychiatric residency programs, they will be more likely to select these alternatives for their training. In the long run, such scientifically trained students who are exposed to a clinically oriented graduate education and given an opportunity to conduct research throughout the educational period may emerge from their training as the scientist-clinicians the field desperately needs.

Another approach is to bring the curricula, students, and faculties of medical and graduate schools closer together. The process begins at the undergraduate level, with interdisciplinary courses that mix students and teachers from many fields and departments to study a common problem. Emerging fields that thrive on this approach, such as biobehavioral science, can and should be encouraged at undergraduate and graduate levels. Another cross-disciplinary stimulus is to allow medical students and psychiatric residents to do graduate work in behavioral science departments; similarly, behavioral science students could benefit from greater access to psychiatry departments, obtaining both their clinical and research experience under psychiatric supervision.

The presence of other behavioral scientists in departments of psychiatry is essential to cross-disciplinary fertilization. They provide psychiatry with the perspective, substance, and methodology of the behavioral sciences and can encourage students in their own disciplines to appreciate the rich store of behavioral science questions to be found in the psychiatric setting.

The education of potential mental health researchers requires that they have role models available whose work they can see, admire, and emulate. This means that psychiatric research personnel in departments of psychiatry and in graduate departments should be available to students at all levels of education. Thus, full-time research should include the invaluable function of teaching—at least to the extent of supervising the elective research of interested students.

The psychiatrist researchers of the next generation will perhaps have been exposed in their undergraduate days to research experience and nurtured in an environment organized frequently by the natural affinity of areas of intellectual endeavor rather than by conventional disciplinary boundaries. As mature scientists, they will still need help in crossing barriers created by scientific specialization and the necessary compartmentalization of knowledge. Thus, it will be important then, as it is now, to encourage extensive interdepartmental collaboration, particularly among clinically oriented psychiatrists and specialists in related basic science disciplines.

Even when psychiatrists are better prepared to conduct their own research and have had more extensive behavioral science backgrounds, the presence of behavioral scientists in departments of psychiatry will continue to be a fertile source of new ideas and theories, as well as a methodological resource.

These suggestions for training research scientists have been based on the assumption that major traditional disciplinary divisions will continue to exist. However, this is not necessarily true or even desirable. For example, one awardee suggested a more radical approach to mental health research education:

> Is there any sentiment toward a more radical reorganization and conceptualization of the training of the advanced-degree mental health professional? Is there something to be gained by evolving toward a dissolution of differences between an M.D. and a Ph.D. in clinical work and making a major effort at emphasizing their common goals? Intuitively I believe there is, after seeing what I think is a marked strain on the university and government resources of supporting two expensive separate disciplines. Also, I think we tend to preserve the M.D.-Ph.D. distinction beyond its usefulness in the mental health field, which may be an increasingly obstructive problem as technology advances. [Then] there is a whole legal problem of licensure. Are we not putting . . . the qualified college under graduate who is becoming dedicated to working in the field of mental health in a ridiculous position of having to choose between two vastly different training philosophies with different interests and legal powers in order to achieve what should be a common body of knowledge and skills? I don't think there is any guarantee that the socially forced differentiation between the M.D. and the Ph.D. adds anything to the self-selected differentiation in these domains that gives variety to approach and leavening of the field. I realize this may have more to do with training than research, but it would advance the whole mental health field by making the major division into research and applied, rather than between M.D. and Ph.D.

The model of the research scientist-clinician who can combine the skills of both approaches is an appealing one for training mental health researchers. Although some feel one person cannot embrace both approaches, Dr. David Shakow, a clinical psychologist and a member of the original Selection Committee for the program, feels it is a useful model. He recently outlined a curriculum he feels is appropriate to educate a mental health research scientist (1971). It assumes that education must be preparation for participating in the widest possible definition of mental health research: "understanding and encouraging potential development in man." He notes that:

> This term "potential" includes for me *both* energies and cognitive capacities. I believe we should be concerned with developing re-

searchers who could be interested in determining man's range of cognitive potential as well as the correlative range of energy potential.

Regarding research attitudes and methodology, Dr. Shakow suggests:

Essentially, it calls for fostering in the student . . . a questioning, critical attitude. . . . This calls for acquisition, among other qualities, of a humility that recognizes how much ignorance characterizes the field.

Dr. Shakow divides his proposed research training program into two parts: substantive and methodological. In the substantive curriculum, he distinguishes knowledge of personality principles, of real-life situations, and of real clinical situations. Methodological study consists of training in specific research techniques and skills, whether these are used to investigate the physiological and behavioral effects of drugs, the processes of adaptation in the neonate, or the cultural origins of destructive attitudes and values.

Regarding methodology, Dr. Shakow believes that training in observation is the general and basic requirement for the mental health researcher. This training must be extensive and rigorous. It must include naturalistic observation, participant observation, "subjective observation" (meaning the empathic skill of responding to cognitive and emotional processes in a subject), and finally self-observation.

When one considers problems of education for psychiatric research, many general questions of purpose and method deserve further exploration; for example:

1. What is the purpose of mental health research?

2. Should training for research be general, specialized, or a mixture?

3. Should plans for the future of psychiatric research involve developing special psychiatric training centers or cultivating those departments that develop competitive strength in research on their own initiative? Or both?

Despite the years of progress in psychiatric research and the success of the Research Development Program in stimulating that progress, psychiatry as a scientific discipline is still in its infancy. Far more questions than answers remain about the nature of mental health and illness. Research has gained a significant toehold in the academic psychiatric community, but its position is still precarious. It will require the full-time, lifetime career commitment of countless talented people to establish that position firmly by producing significant research results.

The experience of the Research Development Program has suggested some productive ways of stimulating research quality and quantity. Ultimately, the future of psychiatric research depends on creating an atmosphere that considers research to be a natural and valued part of the profession. This atmosphere results from the interaction of numerous values and behavior patterns both within and without the profession. Offer, Freedman, and Offer (1972) have described the quality of that interaction:

> At the heart of the matter is the fact that discovery in a vacuum is fruitless. A field is required in which transactions among the generations of teachers, colleagues, students, and patients render ideas viable in the entire process of articulated training, service, and research. These transactions—whatever the gaps in time and fashion —bring research into play with the field and in so doing, if the research can generate interest, change the field. Broadly, the act of inquiry and the valuing of it are of defining importance both to the history of individuals and the profession they claim. . . .
>
> The facts are that communications do actually occur in a community. The community is comprised of those investigators in the biobehavioral sciences relevant to psychiatry, teachers educating the next generations of students, groups and individuals delivering services to the mentally ill, and planners formulating mental health policies and programs. An absorption either in health delivery or in a concern for the resources derived from science tap different personal preferences and evoke varying emphases and values. Yet both interests comprise a part of the total fabric. . . .
>
> Delivering services to the mentally ill is, of course, central. It reflects the nature of the psychiatric obligation to deliver care and to do so in the absence of certain knowledge. However, there is also an obligation to be receptive to knowledge, one that is not always fulfilled. Incorporated within the current retreat from complexity, intellectual challenge, and history is a misrepresentation of research activities as occurring in isolation from modern medical needs or practices. Research is neither alien to nor necessarily competitive with concerns for health delivery. Linkages between research and service occur commonly in medicine—and finally are beginning to occur in psychiatry—as research findings are more widely appreciated and occasionally applied. Ironically, when findings are applied —such as penicillin for syphilis or crisis intervention on the battlefield to prevent shell shock—the origins of such steps in prior inquiry and knowledge are generally promptly forgotten. Nevertheless, there is always a need for a commonality and community of practices and ideas out of which investigative activities are activated and from which they gain both meaning and relevance. Thus, for the life of inquiry, both researchers and an audience of participating students and practitioners are necessary.[1]

[1] Excerpted from *Modern Psychiatry and Clinical Research: Essays in Honor of Roy R. Grinker, Sr.* Edited by Daniel Offer and Daniel X. Freedman. © 1972 by Basic Books, Inc., Publishers, New York. Reprinted by permission.

# History of the Research Development Program

**6**

*The Setting*

The trend toward a more scientific psychiatry now seems to have gathered sufficient momentum to sustain itself. But at the time the Research Development Program was conceived (as the Career Investigator Grant program) in the early 1950s, such a development in psychiatry was perhaps imaginable but hardly to be expected in only 20 years.

At that time, there was almost no scientific research in psychiatry. The typical department of psychiatry was primarily oriented to training for psychiatric practice and was rarely enriched by scientific insights and attitudes, since there was little ongoing departmental research. A few academic departments (probably fewer than 10) were exceptions to the rule, being receptive to the behavioral sciences, pharmacology, and neurosciences, and encouraging research by faculty members, but they were very much a minority vanguard. According to one estimate, there were about two dozen full-time psychiatric researchers in the entire country in the early 1950s.

In the absence of a firm scientific foundation for his practice, even the academic psychiatrist often depended more on faith and a body of clinical experience than on objective knowledge (a situation that is only gradually changing). For many conditions the psychiatrist confronted, treatments were ineffective (although not necessarily recognized as such); when they did work, the relevant therapeutic factors were often unknown.

Psychoanalysis was the dominant theory and in the 1950s was in its heyday, being virtually required training for almost any academically bound psychiatrist, regardless of his career plans as clinician, researcher, or both.

When psychoanalysis emerged as a theory, a method, and a treatment, it came to dominate American psychiatry for good reason. It had, and has, a great deal to offer: a rational account of irrational behavior, a way of thinking and dealing with almost anything a patient did or said, and a rationale for waiting to ascertain the true nature of problems rather than forcing a quick and premature explanation. And people did get better. In short, it was so far superior to anything that had preceded it that it was widely adopted. But the magnitude of the psychiatric problem, combined with physicians' needs to feel competent and confident and the unavailability of alternative methods, led to the tendency to adopt on faith and teach on faith. Utter faith in a system, however understandable and however valuable the system, is nonetheless incompatible with the basic intellectual skepticism required for scientific research. As Asher noted in 1959:

> If you admit to yourself that the treatment you are giving is frankly inactive, you will inspire little confidence in your patients (unless you happen to be a remarkably gifted actor), and the results of your treatment will be negligible. But if you believe fervently in your treatment even though controlled tests show that it is useless, then your results are much better, your patients are much better, and your income is much better, too. I believe this accounts for . . . the violent dislike for statistics and controlled tests that fashionable and successful doctors commonly display [p. 417].

Psychoanalysis, as a particular approach to the treatment of mental and emotional disorder, then as now, has been particularly resistant to the overtures of science, despite considerable good will on the part of psychoanalysts. It was developed and accepted in the context of clinical practice. It is inherent in the theory that one must undergo psychoanalysis before one can understand it at a level that permits meaningful critical evaluation. The number of psychoanalysts who have undertaken a scientific examination of the character, structure, and success of psychoanalysis is very small. As late as 1961, Ham suggested that:

> The relative absence of the type of experimental evidence and quantitative data used in other sciences to validate theories and hypotheses requires students and nonanalytic faculty to accept "on faith" many of the principles taught in these new [psychoanalytic] courses.

Even today, progress in the scientific evaluation of psychoanalytic concepts continues to be exceedingly slow and remains insignificant in comparison to the degree of scientific scrutiny that has been applied to the learning-theory base of behavior therapies or the biochemical base of psychopharmacologic therapy.

Although the growth of psychiatric research had been minimal before the 1950s, several currents combined by the mid-1950s to alter the course of American psychiatry. First, the critical need for new research information was apparent. The supply of psychiatrists was woefully inadequate to meet postwar demands. There was approximately one psychiatrist available for every 1,000 or 10,000 persons who needed his help (the estimates vary according to which definition of mental illness is used). The psychoanalytic approach, consuming seemingly endless man-hours per patient, was neither the most efficient nor the most effective way of coping with demands for treatment. If only on the grounds that therapeutic resources should be made available to all who needed them, the psychoanalytic approach was bound to come under attack or at least be challenged by other approaches to mental illness.

Shepherd (1971) calls 1956 the beginning of the psychiatric revolution because in that year two significantly different papers were presented at the annual meetings of the American Psychiatric Association. At those meetings, Ernest Jones gave what Shepherd calls a hagiographic account of Freud. The following day, Percival Bailey's lecture "concealed a full-scale, erudite, and well-documented attack on the theory and practice of psychoanalysis and its founder."

To show the shift away from an exclusive concern for psychoanalytic theory, Shepherd (1971) cites two statements, 11 years apart, by John Romano, who served as Chairman of the Career Investigator Selection Committee in 1956–1957. In 1950, Romano said that "... psychiatry, particularly through psychoanalytic psychology, will play a major role in the scientific humanization of biology. ..." But by 1961, Romano's tone had changed significantly:

> Though the products of psychoanalytic psychology have been of inestimable value in providing a conceptual frame of mind or mental approach, it obviously cannot serve as a general psychology, much less a satisfactory approach to human biology, exclusive of social concepts [Shepherd, 1971].

To Shepherd, 1956 was a landmark year in the psychiatric revolution also because the importance of psychopharmacology was recognized then in a conference sponsored jointly by the National Institute of Mental Health, the National Academy of Science's National Research Council, and the American Psychiatric Association. The impact of psychopharmacologic developments had already been felt several years earlier.

Before 1950, psychiatry had discovered no drugs of demonstrable importance in affecting mood, thought, and behavior, although there was interest in finding them. In the early 1950s, the discovery that chlorpromazine and reserpine could have a dramatic effect on the course of schizophrenic behavior led to an entirely new field: psychopharmacology. Quite beyond the specific effects and uses of drugs, the advent of psychopharmacology encouraged some profound ongoing changes in psychiatry: it strengthened the growing trend in psychiatry to look outside itself and into the behavioral sciences, both biological and social, for other sources of assistance; it stimulated interest in science as a source of new information that might help treat mental disorder; and it encouraged the study of brain-behavior relations.

The effects of psychopharmacological discoveries are still so new and are developing so rapidly that we cannot assess them yet. However, some of the consequences are already obvious—for example, the significant role of psychopharmacological drugs over the years in reducing the number of patients in our public mental hospitals. Reducing the role of the custodial mental hospital as an institution for handling patients also prompted psychiatry to concern itself further with the character and structure of the community or social milieu in which patients lived, a trend that had been growing since the early 1950s. As psychopharmacology was born of a necessary interaction between the pharmacological scientist and the psychiatric clinician, the broader perspective it stimulated subsequently produced a multidisciplinary interaction of clinician with biochemist, cytogeneticist, pharmacologist, physiologist, psychologist, sociologist, anthropologist, and statistician, among others. Gradually some leaders in psychiatry began to realize that excellence in a clinical facility can be maintained only in an atmosphere of intellectual curiosity and critical appraisal that research stimulates. They had come to the position cited by Shepherd (1971):

> It might be wise to accept the verdict of Rothman that "unless our philosophy of science becomes more critical, experimental, more deductive and inventive, we will remain in the Renaissance period of medical history awaiting a Harvey to catapult us into the Seventeenth Century.

The Research Development Program was initiated by men who recognized that psychiatric research was an essential prerequisite to psychiatric progress. They appreciated the problems that had retarded its development and set out to overcome them. Although we have called the Research Development Program by one general name throughout this book to avoid confusion, actually it has had several names since its inception, reflecting its changing scope and purpose. The following pages will explore the growth and development of the program and how its existence has helped to make the psychiatric revolution more of a reality.

### Career Investigator Grant Program: 1954–1961

The Research Development Program of the National Institute of Mental Health has had three phases. The Research Scientist Development Program (which formally dates from 1967) is the heir to and logical outgrowth of two preceding NIMH programs: the Career Investigator Grant Program (1954–1961) and the NIMH-NIH Research Career Development Program (1961–1967). Despite the administrative changes that necessitated and created these three programs, there has been a remarkable unity of purpose, which is best understood by examining the immediate background, goals, and achievements of the initial NIMH Career Investigator Grant Program.

*The NIMH Background.* In 1946, the National Mental Health Act authorized establishment of the National Institute of Mental Health to carry out a three-fold program of research, training, and service activities related to mental health. The opening sentences of the Act stressed the need to foster "research, investigations, experiments, and demonstrations relating to the cause, diagnosis, and treatment of psychiatric disorders."

At the time, mental health research in the United States, as elsewhere, was diffuse, scattered, and uncoordinated. As mentioned earlier, acute postwar demands for treatment and hospital facilities for the nation's mentally ill, combined with equally acute manpower shortages in the relevant therapeutic professions underscored the need to discover new, more effective methods of prevention and treatment.

The philosophical framework of the NIMH Research Grants and Fellowships Branch Program was set quite early. First, it was recognized that, lacking definite clues to the etiology or best methods of treatment of mental illness, it would be wisest to support the best research in any and all fields related to mental health and illness, whether clinical or nonclinical, basic or applied, empirical, methodological, or theoretical, in the physical, biological, social, or behavioral sciences. Second, NIMH policy over the years had assumed that successful research requires maximum freedom for the researcher. The scientific aims and activities of investigators working under research grants therefore were not to be directed or regimented. The wisdom of this philosophy has been proven repeatedly. Although NIMH did not attempt to direct research or to set rigid research priorities, throughout the history of the grant program, the major emphases implicitly have been to support (1) research on mental illness and the hospitalized mentally ill and (2) basic research (investigations into the process and mechanisms of behavior, whether psychological, social, or biological), which has been viewed as the most effective path to understanding etiology and developing therapeutic and preventive measures.

In 1952, after five years of growth, the NIMH research grant program had spent slightly over $5 million for 165 projects emphasizing the etiology of mental illness, development or evaluation of treatment methods, normal child development, the structure and functions of the nervous system, and the relation of environmental stress to mental health and illness. Psychiatrists and psychologists, who submitted 64 percent of the total applications, were awarded 70 percent of all funds. However, given the lack of a research tradition in psychiatry, many interested research-oriented psychiatrists lacked the training and experience to compete successfully with other applicants.

In 1952, NIMH was considering its recent past and its future. At that time, a moving force was the National Advisory Mental Health Council, consisting of both lay members and outstanding medical and scientific authorities in the study, diagnosis, and treatment of psychiatric disorders. This advisory group was authorized by the National Mental Health Act to make recommendations to the Surgeon General for mental health activities and functions, to review and recommend support for research and training projects, and to collect and make available information on studies in the mental health field. At the November 1952 meeting of the Council, the Council Committee on Review of the NIMH Research Grants (consisting of Dr. William Malamud, Miss Mildred Scoville, and Dr. S. Bernard Wortis) had met with Dr. John C. Eberhart, Chief of the Research Grants and Fellowships Branch of NIMH, and recommended that special research fellowships be made available to help young psychiatrists receive training and engage in research on a relatively long-term basis. They suggested:

> Awards of three to five years duration to provide [annual] stipends of $7,000 to $10,000 for well-trained young investigators, particularly in the field of psychiatry, to enable such men to begin careers of research in well-equipped and well-staffed university departments. Such awards would be similar to those now being made by the Markle Foundation.

The Committee noted that a similar recommendation had also been made by NIH Inter-Council Committee on Institutional Grants. The proposed awards posed some administrative challenges. First, it was not clear that the necessary legislative authorization was available in the fellowship program, which in fact provided for only the standard type of pre- and postdoctoral research fellowship. Second, the money available to the research fellowship program was inadequate to support the new program. In addition, the awards would be unusual in combining characteristics of both research grants and fellowships, providing funds for both training and research. Discussion thus centered on the best administrative mechanism for encouraging superior young scientists to participate in the program. Many of the Council members preferred to view the awards as fellowships. Dr. Ernest Hilgard suggested that since fellowships tend to postpone permanent career decisions and create academic instability, a useful award would be one that would allow younger men to remain on academic faculties, although with lightened loads and great freedom for intellectual exploration. Dr. Eberhart suggested that the five-year fellowships might more effectively stimulate career commitments to research if universities agreed to retain fellows as faculty members at the end of the grant period.

At the request of the Council, Dr. Eberhart and Mr. Philip Sapir subsequently drafted a proposal for awarding what were tentatively called Advanced Research Fellowship Grants. In the discussion that accompanied review of that draft and unanimous approval by the Council, the issue was again raised that the novel program, combining both research and training, was administratively difficult to categorize. (During the program's long history, this characteristic has meant that although it was administered as a type of research grant until 1964, it was subsequently treated as a training program. In March 1964, it was shifted from the NIMH Research Grants Branch to its Training and Manpower Resources Branch, only to return to its original status as a research grant program in March 1973.) Whatever the differing opinions of the Council members concerning the administrative mechanism of dealing with the new awards, they were unanimous about the need for and wisdom of initiating them.

According to Dr. Eberhart, at the time the program was conceived, very few psychiatrists were doing systematic research. As he noted in the June 9, 1953, draft of the program:

> At the present time there are probably fewer than two dozen psychiatrists engaged in full-time research in the United States. Research appointments beyond the post-doctorate fellowship level are so scarce that there is little incentive for the younger man whose talents and interests are in research to plan for this kind of career rather than one in clinical practice or teaching.

The program's originators recognized that young psychiatrists represented a special economic population. Financial rewards were appre-

ciably less for the research psychiatrist than for his clinical colleagues. Although ultimately it would be the man's own intellectual values that would
encourage him to undertake a research career, a relatively well-paying and
long-term program of support might attract the brightest young psychiatrists
into research careers in departments of psychiatry. The hope was that if the
awardees were good enough, medical schools would hire them after the
five-year awards ended. In addition, since many talented young psychiatrists
had had no access during their formative years to scientific role models—
psychiatrists doing full-time research—the program would build a resource
for mental health research in the form of role models for future researchers
to emulate.

As described in a July 1953 memo by Dr. Seymour D. Vestermark,
then Acting Director of NIMH, the new grant, which was approved by Dr.
Robert Felix, Director of NIMH, would differ from ordinary research grants
by being:

> ... an instance of supporting men rather than projects, and a device
> to recruit more able men for research careers in psychiatry and related
> fields. ... These grants are intended to recruit and support able
> younger men, to give them status in good departments while they
> spend essentially full time in research, and to encourage departments
> to appoint such men to their own staff at the termination of the
> grants. Ordinary research grants can support such men but are not
> of much help in recruiting compared to the lucrative possibilities of
> private practice.

The new program was to be administered essentially like other
research grants using the facilities of the Division of Research Grants. For
the first year, the program was expected to provide about five awards (out of
an expected 20 applications) with grants averaging from $12,000 to $15,000
per year. The initial cost would thus be about $60,000 to $75,000 per year.

Since the program was new, approval had to be obtained from
the National Institute of Health. It was general NIH policy to judge innovative programs from the perspective of their potential applicability to all
other institutes. Since at the time NIH was not ready to make the unusual
financing a feature for all institutes, the program was approved as a test
case. If successful, it would later be duplicated NIH-wide. It was.

The program was approved by the Surgeon General prior to the
November 1953 meeting of the Council, and the first announcement of the
new Career Investigator Grant program was sent in 1953 to departments of
psychiatry and psychiatric research institutions. In addition to providing the
grantee with a stipend of from $6,000 to $10,000 for three to five years, the
new grants would include funds "to provide for the costs of his research or

for travel incident to his research or training" as well as an 8 percent indirect-cost reimbursement for the sponsoring institution.

Candidates were also informed that:

> . . . in reviewing applications, the Committee and the Council will be concerned equally with (a) the qualifications of the candidate as demonstrated in part by the nature of the program of research and training for research that he proposes, and (b) the facilities of the institution making the request for providing a stimulating environment for maximum growth of the candidate as a scientific investigator. . . .
>
> Since the shortage of research personnel is greater in psychiatry than in the related basic science disciplines, preference will be given to applications that propose the appointment of a psychiatrist to a research position on the staff of the applicant institution. This does not exclude proposals for the appointment to departments of psychiatry of outstanding young research men from clinical medicine, the biological sciences, or the behavioral sciences. . . .
>
> It is not intended that these grants be used to secure a research man for an institution or department without senior staff competent to advise and guide a young and promising investigator. The National Institute of Mental Health is interested equally in the research to be carried out and in the continued research development of the investigator.
>
> In describing the investigator's responsibilities as "full-time research," there is no desire to prescribe rigidly the program to be followed by him. One or more years of his tenure on the grant may be devoted wholly or partly to training for research in a special area. Such training may be obtained at the host institution or he may spend such time as is needed at one or more institutions. . . .
>
> In addition to research and training for research, the investigator may wish to undertake a small amount of teaching or clinical work as a part of his career development. Such activities would be permitted if he and his sponsor regard them as desirable. The investigator would not be authorized to undertake such nonresearch activities as clinical practice for the sake of additional income, nor would the host institution be permitted to assign to him routine clinical or teaching duties. The basic purpose of the grant, which should not be lost sight of, is to provide the investigator with freedom for research and an opportunity for continued growth as a scientist.

To be eligible for the program, a candidate was required to be a citizen of the United States, to have "demonstrated outstanding promise in research," and to have "completed the usual training in his field":

> For psychiatrists and other physicians, this will ordinarily mean the completion of at least two and preferably three years of residency training. For students in the basic science disciplines, this will mean

at least the completion of doctoral training. It is likely that most candidates will not be more than five years beyond completion of residency training or of the Ph.D.

Candidates were required to apply through a particular department in the institution of their choice, and departments were initially restricted to recommending only one candidate, although this restriction was later waived. The main provisions of the original Career Investigator Grant program are strikingly like those of the present program; in spirit, they are indeed continuous.

By November 1953, the new grant program, called the "Mental Health Career Investigator Grants," had been instituted and grant applications had been received. As the program was initially conceived, applications would be finally reviewed by the National Advisory Mental Health Council, but this body would "place heavy reliance [on a] selection committee composed of present and former Council and Study Section members."

According to Dr. Eberhart, who initially headed the program, the choice of appropriate Selection Committee members was a vital aspect of the program's inception. Since the program essentially provided support for promising young men with ideas rather than their specific research projects, the Selection Committee members needed to be both astute judges of individual character and productive potential as well as critics of scientific merit.

The actual choice of Selection Committee members proved to be felicitous. Dr. Alan Gregg was chosen Chairman. He had been Vice-President for Medical Affairs at the Rockefeller Institute and had worked there for 25 to 30 years; he had extensive experience in spotting talented young scientists for support; Dr. Eberhart called him "the best picker of medical talent." The other outstanding Committee members included Drs. John Benjamin, Professor of Psychiatry, University of Colorado School of Medicine (later Chairman of the Mental Health Study Section); David Shakow, Chief Psychologist, Illinois Neuropsychiatric Institute, Illinois College of Medicine; Horace W. Magoun, Professor of Anatomy, UCLA, and a member of the Council; and Henry W. Brosin, Director of the Department of Psychiatry, University of Pittsburgh.

In January 1954, the Mental Health Career Investigator Selection Committee (as it was officially designated) met with NIMH staff to discuss the function and prospects of the recently announced program. Their judgment expressed both a scientific, professional idealism and an experienced appraisal of scientific status in psychiatry. They hoped, as NIMH Director Dr. Robert Felix put it, that the new program would "give psychiatrists courage to deviate from accepted norms of clinical psychiatry."

They recognized that psychiatric research was restricted in scope and manpower more than research in other medical specialties, and that leadership in psychiatric research was vested mainly in distinguished persons who functioned broadly as psychiatric statesmen and administrators, with full responsibility for clinical services and education as well as for research. Thus, they were united in viewing their most important function as one of encouraging and supporting psychiatrists in research careers.

This primary objective was accepted with awareness of the need for research on psychiatric problems (as distinguished from the need to have psychiatrists in research), and recognizing the essential value of including behavioral scientists from other disciplines in psychiatric research programs. In fact, at the first meeting of the Selection Committee, it was clearly agreed to "encourage collaboration of nonpsychophobic biologists with nonbiophobic psychiatrists," as Dr. John Benjamin put it.

The objectives of research career support, as conceived in 1954, have survived all subsequent changes in program administration. These objectives were: (1) to find promising young psychiatrists, encourage them to undertake and continue with research careers; (2) to provide support for promising young scientists in related disciplines who would work in departments of psychiatry; and (3) also on occasion to support outstanding young investigators in nonpsychiatric disciplines and departments who demonstrate promise of contributing significantly to the mental health field. (The current Research Scientist Development Program fulfills all three goals.)

In 1954, the first of these objectives was an innovation, and the Selection Committee members wondered how to accomplish it. There was no accepted professional model to evaluate, no experience of selection to draw on that seemed to have more than theoretical relevance, and no clear indication of which kinds of psychiatric scientists would be productive, or what talents and training they would require. The resourceful and skilled Committee began with a commitment to clinical insight and dynamic psychiatry, which meant reliance on psychoanalytic training and the grantees' personal qualities of originality, clarity of thought, motivation, and capacity for sustained scientific endeavor.

The original Selection Committee members did not expect, as they looked ahead, studied applications, and interviewed candidates, that most of the psychiatrists whom they would select and support would do well in research, or really become devoted to research careers. Dr. Gregg said that on the basis of experience in England with a comparable type of advanced fellowship program, "a batting average of one in four successful recipients could be considered very good, and an average of 33 1/3 percent successes could be considered phenomenal." All agreed that if one in four were to have productive research careers, the Committee could feel proud of the accomplishment.

Many of the factors militating against a higher success rate were inherent in the organization of the psychiatric profession. Some of these were mentioned more than 12 years later at a meeting of the Northeastern Professors of Psychiatry and members of the NIMH staff administering the Research Career Development Program:

> [The view of department chairmen of] the Research Career Development [Program] awards, as well as of the Career Teacher Awards, is conditioned by the problems that are most difficult in the administration of psychiatric departments. There are not enough teachers of psychiatry employed in university departments. Residents continue to be used to make up deficiencies of the clinical staff. Demands for service continue to exceed possibilities of extending and improving the psychiatric faculty. From this point of view, the psychiatric investigator supported by the Research Career [Development] Program is a very favored person, and he excites some jealousy and resentment. He is not available for continual emergency assignments to clinical work and general psychiatric teaching. The psychiatric investigator, furthermore, is often engaged in laboratory work that appears to be remote from the interests of his colleagues, who are dealing with everyday clinical problems. Thus, although the majority of a group such as the Northeastern Professors would consider that the Research Career Program is valuable and that its purpose, which is to increase the number of psychiatrists engaged in research, is altogether desirable, they would still like to have a group of psychiatric investigators who at the same time function as clinicians and as teachers. . . .

Despite the difficulties facing the pioneer participants in the program, the Committee's expectations proved to be modest: of the first 18 psychiatrists supported by Career Investigator Grants, 12 were found to be functioning influentially as research psychiatrists with national reputations as research scientists when surveyed some 12 to 18 years later; the success rate of two-thirds was more than twice what Dr. Gregg said would be "phenomenal"!

Subsequent discussions by the Selection Committee and relevant NIMH members reveal a second error of their prophetic powers. The group members initially thought that as knowledge of the Career Investigator Grant program spread, applicants in large numbers would request support. The Committee expected to recruit consultants to carry the necessary load of site visits and interviews. By 1956, however, it was clear that no such burden of applications would materialize. Ten applications had been submitted for the first review in January 1954, and in 1956 the number was approximately the same. In fact, a substantial increase did not occur until 1960–1961, the final year of the Career Investigator Grant program. During the seven years of the program, 37 awards were given; 32 to psychiatrists, three to psychologists, and two to nonpsychiatric physicians interested in neuropsychiatry and psychosomatic research. All Career Investigator Grants were awarded to support research in departments of psychiatry or other departments in medical schools or hospitals.

The need for research psychiatrists and for stronger (better organized, broader, more vigorously pursued, and more sustained) research on the problems of clinical psychiatry was perceived not only by the practical idealists on the Selection Committee. Many noted psychiatrists in academic and clinical settings were also strong proponents of the program. Chairmen of leading medical school departments—such as Drs. Fredrick C. Redlich at Yale, Edwin F. Gildea at Washington University, Maurice Levine at Cincinnati, William Malamud at Boston University, and Roy R. Grinker at Michael Reese—supported the program and, when they could, encouraged young staff members to apply. Psychiatrists distinguished in research—Drs. Erich Lindemann at Massachusetts General Hospital, Eli Robins at Washington University, and George Engel at the University of Rochester, for example—also sponsored applicants. Drs. Robert Livingston, Director, Basic Research, NIMH and National Institute of Neurological Diseases and Blindness, Howard Armstrong, Cook County Hospital, Lawrence C. Kolb, Columbia University, and John Romano, University of Rochester, served on the Selection Committee during the early years of the program.

But young men in psychiatry who were prepared and motivated for the unusual commitment of a career of essentially full-time research (at least for five years during a crucial time in personal development) were very rare then, and young women even rarer—as they are even today, when the professional mode of the research psychiatrist has become far more substantially established and tested for security and professional advancement. A balance had to be achieved by the Selection Committee between support of unsystematized though productive endeavors by rare individuals in experimental work and support of ongoing programs of research that could accommodate small or large groups for projects with overlapping requirements, as well as individuals at different levels of experience and competence.

*Review Procedures.* Despite the desire of the Selection Committee to increase the number of scientists engaged in psychiatric research, the members have continually maintained very high standards of quality for potential grantees, their research programs, and the support capacities of their sponsoring institutions.

To assure careful assessment of candidates, the original Selection Committee developed a three-step procedure that has been consistently retained; it consists of preliminary review, site visit, and final review. Through all changes in membership or in responsibility, the Committee has retained its policy to base most award recommendations on information obtained through site-visit interviews with candidates and their sponsors, as well as on the candidates' written proposals (see Appendix C: The Selection Process).

*Training Plans.*   The Selection Committee has always been concerned with plans for candidates' research training as well as for their research. The basic requirement for training has been the availability of an interested senior staff of research scientists. Occasionally, a Career Investigator has served as apprentice to his senior colleagues. Usually, however, the Career Investigator has been relatively independent in his research, and whatever tutoring, supervision, or counsel he received depended on his own sensitivity and initiative.

Until recently, much of the formal training recommended by the Committee for approval has been psychoanalytic. In evaluating requests for this training, the Selection Committee has asked itself whether the candidate's interests in research and his plans for developing an experimental program will be enhanced by acquiring psychoanalytic knowledge and skills. The Committee members have been flexible in interpreting answers to this question. Candidates have not been specifically required to give evidence either that they would test psychoanalytic hypotheses in their own experiments or that they would collect data by psychoanalytic techniques.

*Career Investigator Conferences.*   Another important educational feature of the program has been the series of Career Investigator Conferences, begun in 1957 and continued until today as a means of bringing grantees and program administrators together to share scientific knowledge and exchange views concerning the program. In late 1956 and early 1957, the Selection Committee members (Drs. John Romano, Chairman, S. Howard Armstrong, Jr., Lawrence C. Kolb, David Shakow, Robert B. Livingston, and Mr. Philip Sapir, Executive Secretary) devoted considerable enthusiastic discussion to the idea of setting up an informal two- to three-day voluntary meeting for all currently supported Career Investigators, together with past and present members of the Selection Committee. They saw the meeting as a way to encourage Career Investigators to meet one another, discuss mutual interests and problems, and permit Committee members to become better acquainted with their grantees. The conferences were to provide a basis for mutual discussion of the program's objectives and ways to further research careers.

The first Career Investigator Conference, held in December 1957, consisted of all 16 Career Investigators, five Selection Committee members, five past members, and three Research Grants and Fellowships Branch staff members (including Dr. Boothe, who had recently become Executive Secretary and Administrator of the Fellowship and Career Investigator Program for NIMH, and Mr. Philip Sapir, who had succeeded Dr. Eberhart as Chief of the Research Grants and Fellowships Branch in 1954).

Initially, alumni as well as current grantees and former and current members of the Selection Committee were invited. By 1962, when attendance rose to 59, only current grantees and Committee members were invited. Since 1962, about 35 to 40 Career Investigators (or those with what were later termed "Research Career Development, Group 1 Awards") and five to 10 NIMH staff and Committee members have typically attended these meetings.

The annual Career Investigator Conferences have yielded many benefits. They have given investigators the best possible sounding board for critical analysis of theoretical and technical problems; have enabled group members and their professional colleagues to plan sustained cooperation with other members; have improved morale by allowing each investigator to participate in a lively group of scientists with similar purpose and idealism; and have given members of the Committee an invaluable opportunity to know the awardees and to evaluate the achievements of the program as a whole. They have also established a community of mental health investigators in clinical psychiatry that has been sustained to the present day by these conferences.

The first Career Investigator Conference, like others that followed, alerted program administrators and consultants to problems facing many of the grantees. This feedback has helped to make the program more responsive to the real needs of young scientists engaging in psychiatric research in an environment that is not always optimal and at a time when the science of psychiatry is just gaining acceptance. For example, as the first Career Investigator Conference revealed, most of the scientists felt isolated and alone in their settings. They requested guidance and supervision and needed considerable reassurance that there would be academic positions available to them when they completed the training phase of their grant.

Their isolation appeared to reflect something about the atmosphere and value system of their positions and their profession.

The professional insecurity of awardees has been a constant source of concern to administrators and consultants. Yet the Committee members have continually attempted to avoid an overly paternalistic approach to program participants. As recently as 1969, at the Twelfth Career Investigator Conference, it was reported that the awardees generally wanted more feedback during the five-year period. They felt very insecure, particularly as they reached the end of the award period, because renewal was uncertain. Committee members reminded the group that NIMH is a granting agency and not a consulting or policing body, and that there were dangers in becoming too paternalistic. They encouraged each individual to assume more responsibility for his own career.

*Strengthening Academic Ties.* In general, program staff and Committee members have attempted to create a more secure atmosphere for grantees by strengthening the ties between the sponsoring institution and the grantee rather than by excessive involvement on the part of the agency itself. Thus, in reviewing applications, Committee members have followed closely several policies designed to create those ties. For example, the eligibility requirements state that preference be given to candidates whose salaries had been paid from temporary funds and to candidates for whom awards would provide the opportunity to spend a major part of their time in research. Interpreting these eligibility requirements strictly, the Committee members have frequently declared applications unacceptable because the award requested would not have benefited the candidate or relieved him f om extensive nonresearch activities.

The Committee members have considered it important to appraise not only the candidate's promise as a research scientist but also the nature of the position to be supported. Applications have thus also been rejected because the Committee found that the arrangement between the candidate and the senior staff of the sponsoring department would not insure good working relations between the awardee and his colleagues and a positive reception of his contributions to the departmental program. By following these policies, the Committee has avoided making program participants appear to be federal rather than institutional employees. It has made every effort to secure assurances from the sponsoring institutions that awardees would enjoy all the rights and privileges of other faculty members, including promotions and tenure decisions. To the extent that future predictions could be made and awardees have maintained the quality of their work, institutions have committed themselves to retaining the investigators on their staffs when award support ended.

Looking back at the initial Career Investigator Grant program as a whole, over its seven-year span from 1954 to 1961, it has had a high rate of success in encouraging high-caliber scientists to engage in psychiatric research. A combination of factors such as the prospective candidates' own choice of a research career, the necessity for institutional sponsorship, and the process of careful, personalized screening of applicants has probably helped this pioneering venture to succeed.

Yet if one studies, as Dr. Boothe did, the progress of the first group of 18 psychiatrists supported by the Career Investigator Grants through 1961, it is obvious that success did not come easily. At the beginning of their Career Investigator support, these psychiatrists had, on the average, more experience than subsequent awardees: five of them had completed (or all but completed) psychoanalytic training, two had graduate degrees in psychology, and four had several years of previous experience in research.

Despite their relative maturity, these first 18 awardees experienced frequent problems (many of which still persist). There was often a struggle to obtain training—theoretical, methodological, and technical—for research in a chosen field. For some, sponsors proved to be elusive, interested in different areas, or with competence that was not relevant to the grantee. For others, departmental clinical services proved to be rigidly indifferent to their needs and requests. For still others, the demands of their psychoanalytic training precluded travel to distant research facilities for extended training. Given these and other problems, many doubted whether a psychiatrist could maintain his identity as a researcher. Indecision about the direction of their professional lives haunted some grantees for several years. It was tempting to retain the possibility of returning to clinical practice (especially on the full-time plan) or to a balanced program of administration, teaching, and practice as an alternative to continuing in research and possibly facing the financial handicaps and insecurity that the researcher often meets. For some, indecision stimulated introspection about personal talents and values: Am I really a scientist or am I essentially a clinician? Is science a personal indulgence at my family's expense?

Impressive, indeed, to those who could observe and sympathize with the Career Investigators in the 1960s were the resourcefulness and resolution by which most of them gained sophistication in research and achieved the necessary local as well as national support for continuing their projects.

As indicated earlier, despite many obstacles and moments of indecision among members of this ground-breaking group, 12 to 18 years after they entered the program, a significant majority had committed themselves to careers as research scientists, as the following figures show:

Continuing in essentially full-time research                              9
Departmental chairmen, half-time in research                              2
Part-time research, with teaching and clinical practice in
    mainly academic settings                          2
Clinical practice, with a secondary research interest                     1
Did not continue in research                                              4
                                                                       18

Of the nine in essentially full-time research, two were mainly involved in directing complex research organizations; seven had continued with a major commitment to experimental projects.

From 1954 to 1961 the Career Investigator Grant program proved its merit in stimulating psychiatrists to undertake research careers. In 1961 the time was ripe to expand the program to provide continuity of support and to reach a wider segment of the growing community of scientists interested in mental health research.

### Research Career Development Program: 1961–1967

In late 1959 and early 1960, the Mental Health Career Investigator Grant Committee prepared a recommendation, supported by the National Advisory Mental Health Council at its March 1960 meeting, to extend the Career Investigator Grant program to include awards for fully qualified investigators. The scope of research to be supported by the program would be broadened, and those who had completed the initial award f ᵣ research and related training could continue with a full-time research commitment.

Since several other NIH Institutes had recommended similar types of programs, and since the initial experience of the Career Investigator Program had been positive, Dr. James A. Shannon, Director of NIH, encouraged planning of an overall NIH research career program. The new NIH Research Career Development Program was announced in October, 1960, and given Congressional endorsement in 1961.

The new NIMH-NIH program had three awards:

A. *Research Career Development Awards:* Five-year awards for young scientists, renewable for an additional five years.

    *Group 1:* For scientists (usually psychiatrists) who need additional research training and a chance to engage in three to five years of full-time research.

    *Group 2:* For independent investigators of more or less limited experience who still need to develop their full potential in research.

B. *Research Career Awards:* Indefinitely renewable awards to provide stable positions enabling experienced investigators to continue productive careers in research and teaching. Intended
to continue through the full professional career of the individual as long as he and the institution wish to continue.
Noncompetitive review every five years. Normally for outstanding investigators under 45 years of age.

The Research Career Development Program marked a significant
step forward from the initial concept of an advanced fellowship providing a
limited stipend, to the concept of a subsidy to an institution for a staff
position with full salary and fringe benefits as determined by the salary scale
of the institution. According to a 1969 review of the NIH program's history:

> For the first time, as a principal program objective, NIH funds
> were used to provide salary stability for scientists engaged in careers
> in biomedical research as members of nonfederal organizations. It
> had become increasingly evident to qualified observers of govern-
> ment-science relationships that expansion of research programs in
> the national interest would require the federal government not only
> to support the training of greater numbers of young developing
> scientists who would pursue research careers, but also to contribute
> toward adequate salary support for the established biomedical in-
> vestigator. The immediate and expeditious way to do this was to
> include funds for salary support as an integral part of federal research
> grants or contracts. This practice was adopted eventually on a large
> scale and even now constitutes a significant mechanism for salary
> support of investigators in nonfederal laboratories. . . . An important
> objective of the program was to strengthen research institutions
> while providing stable support to individuals. To provide a con-
> tinuing link between the individuals selected and their institutions,
> a number of ties to the institution were preserved under the pro-
> gram. Awardees were expected to participate in the general activities
> of the institution, including [a minimal amount of] teaching. Awards
> were not made to individuals but were made to institutions on behalf
> of individuals. The NIH award was consistent with the salary scale
> of the institution for persons with comparable experience and ac-
> complishments. Finally, the institution was asked to nominate for
> [the senior] Career Awards only those whom it would wish to have
> as permanent staff. Taken together, it was expected that these pro-
> visions would link the institution and the awardees effectively under
> a program for which salaries were provided by a federal agency.

The NIMH Research Career Development Program was administered in close cooperation with the Career Development Review Branch
of the NIH Division of Research Grants. A special feature of the NIMH
program, as distinguished from the Research Career Development Program

in other Institutes, was the provision of a research grant, not to exceed $5,000 annually, for investigators with the Research Career Development, Group 1 Award who did not have other research support. Applications for these research grants were reviewed by the Research Career Award Committee and evaluated in relation to the research proposals contained in the career program applications. For most of the younger investigators, the amount provided for research projects proved sufficient. Some who needed funds for expensive research projects applied successfully for larger research grants through the regular research grant program of NIH.

The majority of investigators with Research Career Development Group 2 or Research Career Awards (for the senior investigators) were also receiving support for actual research costs through regular research grants, which they obtained by standard procedures. In a small number of cases at the Group 2 level, usually when an award enabled an investigator to undertake a new position without support from an ongoing regular research grant, adjunctive research grants up to $10,000 per year (and limited to a two-year period) were awarded, thus enabling the investigator to finance experimental work at the beginning of a Research Career Development Program award, pending support from a regular research grant.

Another special feature of the NIMH Research Career Development Program reflected the desire of NIMH to continue, in the Group 1 award, the special training feature of the earlier Career Investigator Grant Program. Authorization was secured from NIH to continue to provide funds for special training costs. Periods of work and formal study in centers away from the sponsoring institutions were encouraged, and tuition fees for course work in other departments were provided, as well as funds for psychoanalytic training costs (in those cases where such training was justified as essential to the substantive aspects of the awardee's proposed research). Candidates were encouraged to propose reasonable plans for their own development. These plans took many forms. One investigator spent a year at NIMH, while another spent two years at the Max Planck Institute in Munich. Several awardees studied at the Brain Research Institute at UCLA, while other young investigators studied abroad, with Drs. Jean Piaget in Geneva, Michel Jouvet in Lyon, France, Richard Jung in Freiburg, John Bowlby in London, and Lawrence Weiskrantz at Oxford. Collaborative arrangements between departments of psychiatry and other departments, such as psychology, medicine, pediatrics, and pharmacology, have also proved to be effective. For the most part, however, the statement of sponsors that training support would be made available to the young investigator, and the grantee's statement of his intentions, were accepted without much critical appraisal. Later, in 1967, when a considerable change in program administration occurred, it seemed reasonable to require a more systematic training plan in the written application and to assess the proposed plan during the initial review and site visit before making an award.

In 1961, when the Research Career Development Program was initiated, the Committee was expanded from its five-man membership to a body of nine, with additional strength in the areas of biochemistry, the social sciences, and psychology. Its membership included representatives from psychiatry, psychology (experimental, neuropsychology, personality-clinical, and developmental), sociology, neurochemistry, psychopharmacology, statistical methods, and research design.

As the program grew, the Committee, which initially had convened only once yearly, began to meet three times a year. From the beginning, in reviewing applications, the site visit has been used extensively. As the review procedure evolved, during a preliminary review, evidence provided by a written application was evaluated and questions for a more searching inquiry were defined. In a subsequent meeting, final review took place and additional evidence from site visits was presented. For Career Development Group 1 awards, site visits were always made. Career Development Group 2 awards were occasionally recommended on the basis of the written application alone if the applicant was well known to the Committee members. (For further discussion of this process, see Appendix C: The Selection Process.)

In 1965, for the first time, the Committee undertook the task of reviewing applications for the renewal of awards originally made at the Group 2 level. Painstaking discrimination was needed, since criteria for renewal included such evidence of continued research promise as productivity, expansion of experimental projects, and improved focus or depth in the conceptualization of the research. Again, site visits proved invaluable. Renewal applications were more frequently recommended for approval than initial award applications; the Committee members averaged a 71 percent approval rate for renewals, compared to their approximately 50 percent approval rate for new applications. The Committee members (most of whom had not been members when the initial awards were made), felt that the highly screened applicants who had won competitive awards five years earlier had usually maintained high-caliber work that deserved continuing support.

As the new, jointly sponsored NIMH-NIH program took shape, the middle-stratum Group 2 awards came to constitute the strongest part of the program, at least in the extent and variety of research being produced. With this award, the NIMH was able to extend mental health research wherever promising investigators needed support for the unrestricted development of their research interests. Awards were available at the Group 2 level for highly qualified psychologists, anthropologists, sociologists, pharmacologists, and specialists in other disciplines working in the departments of graduate schools, mental health institutes affiliated with medical schools, schools of social work, general hospitals, and other centers.

Although the Group 2 program grew rapidly to have the largest number of awardees of the three groups, the Group 1 award (comparable to the earlier Career Investigator Grant and granted to the 37 original awardees who had been in the earlier program) was considered by the program administrators and Committee members to represent the heart of the program. The award for the psychiatrist at the beginning of his research career had always enjoyed the highest priority in the esteem of the consultants and staff (a status officially acknowledged when in February 1964 the Committee, in response to a request by the Associate Director of NIH for Training Programs, assigned priorities to the three types of awards and gave first priority to the Group 1 award).

These priorities may be better understood if two of the program's objectives are considered: (1) to find and support promising psychiatrists who are willing to enter upon careers of research; and (2) to improve the quality of psychiatric research and make it more productive. Since the second objective depends mainly on success of the first, the major investment in the administration of the program has been directed to the more basic award.

The third type of award, the Research Career Award, has held a tenuous place in the history of the program. It was created to allow distinguished scientists to devote full time to research and related activities and to pursue theoretical and scholarly leads as well as experimental objectives—a freedom still rare in mental health research. The awards were given at about the same rate as the Group 1 Awards during the first three years of the program (1961–1964). However, as the total NIH Research Career Development Program grew rapidly in costs, doubling the number of NIH-wide awardees (from 127 to 262) between 1962 and 1964, NIH officials became seriously concerned with increasing long-term funding requirements and program costs. This was especially true in view of steady tightening and reapportioning of NIH training grant funds. Thus, a thorough re-evaluation and reconsideration was given to all aspects of the program. As a result, in June 1964, the authority to make new indefinitely renewable Research Career Awards was discontinued (although all active current Research Career Awards were continued under the terms and conditions of the original award). The NIMH program thus had no provision for support of senior investigators beyond the developmental levels.

Among the reasons for eliminating new Research Career Awards throughout the various institutes of NIH were the following: there was a danger that an indefinitely renewable award without competitive review might support an investigator who would become nonproductive; some research career awards had been provided for scientists who already had adequate support for essentially full-time research; some institutions did not approve of the support of professorships by federal funds and with the stipulated conditions of the Research Career Awards; some investigators with Research Career Awards tended to play federal support against the authority of the sponsoring institution; and, finally, continuation of the Research Career Program would result in too great an expenditure.

After the senior-level Research Career Awards were closed to new applicants, NIMH personnel attempted repeatedly to find an alternative method to support the senior scientists. From 1964 until 1967, the National Advisory Mental Health Council frequently voiced its concern about this lack of continuity, particularly as awardees approached the end of the maximum support available (two five-year terms) by Research Career Development Awards.

The NIMH program directors ultimately put forth the terms of a revised program which was, in 1967, to become known as the Research Scientist Development Program of NIMH, to be administered independently from the Research Career Development Program of NIH.

### Research Scientist Development Program: 1967–1973

The NIMH Research Scientist Development Program, established in 1967, represented the culmination of over 12 years of experience in sponsoring research training and experience for scientists conducting mental health research. In many respects, it resembled the original design of the Research Career Development Program. There were two types of five-year, renewable Research Scientist Development awards for the younger scientist: Type I (like the earlier Group 1), offering training in addition to a salary for research experience, and Type II (like Group 2), offering a salary for research. Awards for the senior scientist (formerly the Research Career Awards) were reinstated under the title "Research Scientist Award." The new program incorporated several changes designed to prevent and circumvent some of the problems that had arisen with the Research Career Award.

The Research Scientist Development Type I award, available for five years, was renewable for another five as a Type II award after competitive review. (A $5,000 research cost allowance was provided in addition to the training allowance.) For Research Scientist Development Type II grantees, the five-year salary awards could be renewed, following competitive review, for one five-year period. (In addition to their salaries, Type II grantees could receive, in unusual circumstances, adjunctive research grants of $10,000 for a maximum of two years.)

The major difference between the new program and its predecessor was in the award for the senior scientist. The earlier Research Career Award recipients had been given essentially lifetime (indefinitely renewable) support, whereas Research Scientists received a five-year award, renewable, after competitive review, for a maximum of 15 years. (The original group of Research Career Award recipients was maintained and supported, however, according to the initial terms of their grants.)

In the policy statements of September 1, 1967, and September 1, 1969, which described the Research Scientist Development Program, several requirements designed to strengthen the bonds between awardee and institution were made explicit. As the early years of the Research Career Award program experience had revealed, a previously established salary limit of $25,000 per year was unrealistic; thus, since 1969 the Research Scientist Development Program had allowed institutions to supplement salaries from nonfederal funds "in amounts compatible with the institutional salary scale."

Although the Research Scientist Development Program awardees were permitted to engage in a limited clinical practice, their fees were to be given to their grantee institution to be used for research and training costs. Under the program's provisions, awardees were to be freed by their institutions to do essentially full-time research:

> The eligibility requirement is that the award would benefit the candidate by:
> a. Relieving him from support by an income derived primarily from research grants, contracts, or similar sources of relatively short-assured duration;
> b. Changing the terms of his current position from a major involvement in the activities other than research to essentially full-time in research; or
> c. Enabling him to accept a new position, in research, for which institutional funds would not be available.

The institutions were expected to create a reasonably secure position for the awardee:

> It is expected that each candidate nominated will be of such quality that the institution would assure him of a continuing position within the financial and legal capacity of the institution to make future commitments.

Despite the requirement that awardees be freed for full-time research, the program policy statement explicitly recognized that participation in many professional activities of awardees' respective institutions was not only inevitable but desirable:

> A scientist supported by the program is professionally responsible to his own institution. His status, title, salary, and staff privileges (including official [leave] and sick leave) are determined by his institution according to its established policies, as adjusted to the requirements of the program. Awards are provided for scientists who devote essentially full time to experimental and scholarly research and related activities, including research training or directing research training. It is not the intention of the National Institute of Mental Health, however, to restrict research scientists from appropriate participation in the activities of their departments. Contributions of research scientists to teaching or clinical programs are recognized as desirable, as [are] contributions to administrative planning or direction. Substantial administrative responsibilities, however, are regarded as inappropriate for scientists supported by the program.

A significant difference between the Research Scientist Development Program of NIMH and the Research Career Development Program (as it was simultaneously continued at NIH) concerned the age of candidates. The NIH Research Career Development Program award was given for five years only to scientists under 40 years of age; initially they could be renewed for a total of eight years but only until the awardee reached 45 years of age. (In 1972, no renewals beyond the initial five years of support have been available in the NIH program.) The NIMH program, in contrast, had no age restriction for any level of award, although the Research Scientist Development, Type I award was understood to be given usually to the youngest scientists (at least three years past their graduate degree), and the Research Scientist Awards were usually given to the most mature scholars.

*Research Development Program Conferences.* The tradition of innovation that has characterized the Research Development Program since its beginnings as the Career Investigator Grant program has been upheld in recent years with the inception of the NIMH Research Development Program Conferences. They were begun in 1968 as a means of encouraging awardees with common research interests (though different disciplinary approaches) to explore, together with nongrantee experts, current findings and problems, future issues, and new directions in their field of inquiry. The 1969 Conference on the Biochemistry of Sleep, for example, was attended by 14 awardees at all levels of the program working in the areas of sleep, brain chemistry, and neuroregulatory processes related to sleep states. Eight invited guests as well as NIMH staff and a Review Committee member also attended.

Unlike most conferences, most of the two-day meeting was devoted to informal discussion rather than to formal papers. According to one of the invited nonawardee participants:

> Several themes emerged at this unique conference (unique particularly due to the high caliber and widely divergent representation of disciplines) that could be characterized as both remarkable happenstances of cross-fertilization and confrontation between scientists working with the brain. It appeared to be a most productive clash of cultures. Each participant had to open his eyes to other ways of thinking than usually encouraged by his particular group of origin. At the same time, each scientist was forced to back off and re-examine his own givens and make explicit previously elided assumptions underlying his own approach. . . .

This participant described the intellectual volleyball of the interdisciplinary conferees during the discussions:

> This kind of weaving from behavior in man to mechanisms of drug action and brain electrical changes to brain neuro-chemistry produced a remarkable scientific counterpoint generating a multitude of new research ideas. New research approaches were spawned relative to such diverse questions as: How do amphetamines work? What relationship exists between chemical mechanisms underlying dreaming and those underlying either drug-induced or naturally occurring psychoses? What techniques are available for more specifically altering brain-chemical information transfer? Might certain known effective anti-psychotogens act as "false brain messengers"?
>
> It is hard for me to imagine a more valuable experience for us and our research.

*The 1972 Program: Award Distribution.* The Research Scientist Development Program and its predecessors have supported 324 scientists between 1954 and 1972, of whom 176 were awardees in 1972. Of the four types of awards given in 1972 (Type I, Type II, Research Scientist Awards, and a continuation of the Research Career Awards for those who received them prior to 1964), the Development Type II (like the earlier Group 2) comprised the largest group (70). Following closely were the Research Scientist Awards (63). This latter group grew rapidly, more than doubling since the initial 28 awards were made in 1968. This growth (which is all the more striking since the other groups' size diminished somewhat since 1968) reflects the use of this level of award to continue support after an awardee has completed 10 years of research experience through Development Awards.

What are the departmental affiliations of awardees? The July 1972 NIMH statistics show that of the 176 awardees at that time, the majority (124) were sponsored by medical school departments. Of these, 78 percent (96) were in departments of psychiatry. Among the 52 awardees in nonmedical departments (for example, academic graduate and research departments), more than half (31) were in departments of psychology.

For most types of awards, there have been significantly more grantees in psychiatry departments than in all other departments—medical or nonmedical. This is most dramatic in the case of the Type I awards, for which (true to the intent of its predecessor, the Career Investigator Grants program) 20 of the 25 awardees were in psychiatry departments. There is, however, an exception: of the 18 Research Career Awards in 1972, 10 awardees were scientists in psychology departments, while four were in departments of psychiatry and another four were in departments of social science, anthropology, and animal behavior.

Comparing the award patterns in medical and nonmedical departments, the Type II award was the most common among medical departments (54 of the 124 awards), while the Research Scientist Award was most common among nonmedical departments (18 of the 52 awards).

Although awardees were primarily in departments of psychiatry, they were not primarily psychiatrists; in fact, of the awardees in 1972, less than one-third were psychiatrists. By far the leading discipline has been psychology, which had 68 grantees. (The third-ranking discipline, pharmacology, had only 13 awardees.)

Among the psychiatrists, Type I Awards have slightly exceeded Type II and Research Scientist Awards (18, 15, and 15, respectively); for psychologists, the Research Scientist Award has been predominant, alone supporting almost half (31) of the 68 psychologists in 1972.

Considering the kinds of research problems studied by awardees of various disciplines, most of the work has been concentrated in two large areas: one might be called neurosciences, and the other is psychology (including comparative, developmental, experimental, personality and experimental psychopathology, and math and statistics).

Research into traditional "psychiatric" problems per se occupied only 13 of the 1972 awardees, of whom 12 were psychiatrists and one a psychologist. About three-quarters of the psychiatrists were conducting research in areas outside their traditional training. Almost all of these were working in neuroscience areas, with seven doing pharmacological research and another four conducting essentially psychological studies. By contrast, almost half (33) of the 68 psychologists were conducting studies in their own field. Scientists in other disciplines were almost all conducting studies in their own disciplines.

In certain areas of study, such as one embracing neuropsychology, psychophysiology, and developmental psychobiology, both psychiatrists and psychologists participated about equally. This was also true of pharmacological areas.

Where are the awardees located? As of July 1972, awards were being given to grantees at 38 medical schools and centers, 39 graduate schools, and four other research institutions throughout the United States. Among the medical institutions there were 124 awards, with all but 11 schools having several awardees. Those with the highest numbers of awardees included Harvard University (12), University of Chicago (8), University of California at Los Angeles (7), University of Colorado (7), New York University (7), Yale University (7), Stanford University (6), and Washington University (6). Thus the program has been fulfilling one of its major goals—to establish a research base in psychiatry departments by building up a nucleus of key researchers in various centers.

The 44 awards to graduate schools were more evenly distributed than those to medical schools. Only one university had more than two awardees: Rutgers University had three at New Brunswick and four at Newark. Universities with two awards were the University of Colorado, Harvard University, University of Illinois, Massachusetts Institute of Technology, University of Michigan, University of Minnesota, University of Missouri, University of Nevada, and University of Wisconsin.

Among the eight awardees at four research institutions that were neither medical nor graduate schools, the Research Center for Mental Health (New York University) had four awardees, and the Institute for Social Research (University of Michigan) had two.

In summary, the Research Scientist Development Program, which has essentially stabilized its growth over the past few years, now supports primarily psychologists and psychiatrists to conduct research in a variety of disciplinary areas, most of which are related to the neurosciences. Medical schools receive slightly more awards than graduate schools. The latter tend to have only one awardee per sponsoring school, while medical schools tend to have more than one.

*Program Growth Trends.* Comparing the Research Scientist Development program with the Career Investigator Grant from which it developed reveals trends in how the program has grown—in numbers of awardees and institutions, in types of disciplines and departments supported, and in the geographical distribution of awards. In the mid 1950s, upper East Coast institutions dominated psychiatric research; nine of the first 23 Career Investigator Awards were sponsored in Boston, three others were also in the Northeast, and four others were no further removed than Pittsburgh, Philadelphia, and Baltimore. By now this dominance has been challenged by increasingly competent departments throughout the country. Although East Coast institutions still receive half of the awards, they are now joined by institutions in the Western, Southern and Central states.

The program has also grown in its breadth of support, encompassing now not only the young psychiatrist-investigator who needs further training but also more experienced research scientists from a host of other behavioral, biological, pharmacological, and neuroscience disciplines. There has been a corresponding shift in emphasis over the years toward the biological sciences and neurosciences as areas of study, even by psychiatrists and psychologists. Accordingly, there has been an emphasis on formal study of research methodology and content in specific areas of scientific interest. The program's sponsors have always encouraged and welcomed clinical research studies and considered them with great favor. Nonetheless, the exciting developments in the neurosciences during the past two decades, and the hope and promise of dramatic new clinically applicable techniques and methods arising from this avenue of research have captured the imagination of young and older scientists alike. Hopefully, in the future, the growing multifaceted attack on the underlying causes of mental illness will yield both an invaluable store of information and the means to prevent and alleviate many of the illnesses that now confront, but confound, psychiatry. It is to that ultimate end that the program has always been dedicated.

# Appendix A: Awardees of the Research Development Program and Their Areas of Study as of March 1, 1973

Ader, Robert, Ph.D., *Psychosomatic Phenomena in Animals*     1964*

Aghajanian, George K., M.D., *Psychotogenic Drug Action on Chemically Defined Neurons*     1965

Ames, Adelbert, III, M.D., *Metabolism and Function in Central Nervous System*     1956†

Anagnoste, Berta F., M.D., *The Effects of Centrally Acting Drugs on Biogenic Amines*     1970

Anders, Thomas F., M.D., *Environment and Maturation in Infant Sleep and Development*     1969–1972

Anderson, Kenneth V., Ph.D., *Neural Mechanisms in Sensory Perception*     1968

Appel, James B., Ph.D., *Psychotomimetic Drugs, Amines, and Behavior*     1969–1972

Aronson, Harriet, Ph.D., *Patient Variables Related to Initiation of Treatment*     1963–1968

Auerbach, Arthur H., M.D., *Patient Responses in Relation to Therapist Behavior*     1964–1969

Axelrod, Seymour, Ph.D., *Neuropsychological Studies of Perception*     1965–1970

Baekeland, Frederick, M.D., *Functional Aspects of Slow-Wave and REM Sleep*     1964

* Date indicates original year of award. When awards have terminated, the final year is indicated as well.

† Indicates original award was a Career Investigator Grant.

Baldessarini, Ross J., M.D., *Synaptic Transmitters in the CNS* — 1970

Baldwin, Alfred L., Ph.D., *Cognitive Development and Cognitive Socialization* — 1964–1969

Baraona, Enrique, M.D., *Mechanism and Complications of Alcoholic Hyperlipemia* — 1972

Barchas, Jack D., M.D., *Neuroregulatory Agents and Behavior* — 1969

Barker, Roger G., Ph.D., *Studies in Psychological Ecology* — 1963–1971

Barnet, Ann B., M.D., *EEG-AER Correlates of Perceptual-Cognitive Development* — 1970

Barondes, Samuel H., M.D., *Biochemical Regulatory Mechanisms and Memory Storage* — 1967–1969

Barry, Herbert, III, Ph.D., *Psychopharmacological Study of Chronic Stressors* — 1967

Bartoshuk, Alexander, Ph.D., *Differential Study of Sensory Activation* — 1964–1969

Bateson, Gregory, M.A., *Communication Processes* — 1964–1970

Bernstein, Stephen, Ph.D., *Neurophysiology of Information Processing in Insects* — 1966

Blacker, Kay H., M.D., *Monitoring Cognition in Mental Patients* — 1964–1969

Blank, Marion S., Ph.D., *Growth of Cognition and Behavior in Early Childhood* — 1965

Block, James D., Ph.D., *Psychophysiological Studies of Autonomic Function* — 1961–1967

Block, Jeanne H., Ph.D., *A Developmental Study of Ego and Cognitive Development* — 1968

Blumenthal, Monica D., M.D., Ph.D., *Biochemical Parameters in Schizophrenia* — 1962–1968

Board, Francis A., M.D., *Psychosomatic Studies of Adaptation to Life Stress* — 1955–1958†

Borowitz, Gene H., M.D., *Psychophysiologic Studies in Anxiety* — 1962–1966

Bossom, Joseph, Ph.D., *Neural and Behavioral Analysis of Visuomotor Plasticity* — 1965–1970

Bourne, Lyle E., Jr., Ph.D., *Development and Use of Logico-Conceptual Rules* — 1971

Bowden, Douglas McH., M.D., *Non-Human Primate Models of Behavior Disorders* — 1970

Brackbill, Yvonne, Ph.D., *Infant Behavior* — 1964

Brady, John Paul, M.D., *Drug-Aided Deconditioning
Treatment of Inhibition*                                      1964
Bridger, Wagner H., M.D., *Determinants of Sensori-
Motor and Cognitive Functions*                               1958†
Brush, F. Robert, Ph.D., *Pituitary-Adrenal Hormones
and Aversive Motivation*                                     1968–1971
Bucher, M. Rue, Ph.D., *Mechanisms of Professional
Socialization*                                               1965–1969
Burke, Cletus J., Ph.D., *Mathematical Psychology*           1963–1973
Buschke, Herman, M.D., *Retention in and Retrieval from
Immediate Memory*                                            1964–1969
Bush, Marshal, Ph.D., *Reality Attentiveness and Selective
Attention*                                                   1971
Byck, Robert, M.D., *Reversible Cold Block in Nervous
System*                                                      1967–1969
Callaway, Enoch, III, M.D., *Relation of Autonomic
Activity to Perception*                                      1954–1958†
Camp, Bonnie W., Ph.D., M.D., *Therapeutic Programs
for Learning Disorders*                                      1972
Carr, Herman E., M.D., *Endocrine Function and Behavior*     1963–1968
Chapman, Loren J., Ph.D., *A Search for Subvarieties of
Schizophrenia*                                               1970
Chapman, Loring F., Ph.D., *Implanted Electrode Studies
in Man*                                                      1964–1965
Chosy, Julius J., M.D., *Psychophysiology of Manifest
Anxiety and Vasovagal Fainting*                              1964–1969
Cicero, Theodore J., Ph.D., *Neurochemical Correlates
of Drug Addiction in Animals*                                1972
Clark, Fogle C., Ph.D., *Experimental Analysis of Operant
Discrimination*                                              1967–1972
Clark, Lincoln, M.D., *Comparative Behavior and Psy-
chopharmacology*                                             1961
Clark, Rita W., M.D., *Origins and Development of
Differentiation*                                             1966–1969
Clayton, Raymond B., Ph.D., *Steroids, Terpenoids, and
Behavioral Biology*                                          1970
Cobb, Sidney, M.D., *Psychosocial Epidemiology*              1963
Colby, Kenneth M., M.D., *Computer Simulation of
Belief Systems*                                              1967
Cole, Michael, Ph.D., *Ontogeny of Learning Components
of Avoidance*                                                1969–1970

Conners, C. Keith, Ph.D., *Drug Effects on Learning and Cortical-Evoked Potentials in Children*                 1969

Cook, Stuart W., Ph.D., *Modification and Measurement of Racial Attitudes*                 1969

Curtis, George C., M.D., *Humoral Patterns and Their Psychological Correlates*                 1961–1966†

Cytryn, Leon, M.D., *(1) Affective Disorders in Childhood; (2) Children with Down's Syndrome*                 1968

Dahl, Hartvig A., M.D., *Quantitative Methods for Studying Psychoanalysis*                 1967–1972

Davis, James A., Ph.D., *Techniques of Survey Analysis*                 1965–1967

Davis, Roger E., Ph.D., *Environmental Control of Memory Formation*                 1968

Davis, Roger T., Ph.D., *Perception by Sub-Human Primates*                 1965–1970

Dement, William C., M.D., Ph.D., *The Nature and Function of REM Sleep*                 1965

Denney, D. Duane, M.D., *(1) CNS Function and Behavior; (2) Factors Leading to Psychiatric Consultation*                 1964–1968

Dewson, James H., Ph.D., *Central Mechanisms in Audition*                 1965–1969

Dohrenwend, Bruce P., Ph.D., *Social Status and Psychological Disorder*                 1971

Douglass, William A., Ph.D., *Strategy Formation in Response to Rapid Social Change*                 1971

Drum, David E., M.D., Ph.D., *Biochemical Properties of Human Liver Metalloenzymes*                 1972

Dulit, Everett P., M.D., Ph.D., *Abstract Thinking in Gifted Adolescents*                 1962–1967

Dunmore, Charlotte J., Ph.D., *Black Children and Their Families*                 1971

Dykman, Roscoe A., Ph.D., *Children with Specific Learning Disabilities*                 1961–1972

Egger, M. David, Ph.D., *Reflex Patterning—In Vivo Microscopy of the CNS*                 1969

Eichler, Myron, M.D., *Altered Biochemical Pathways and Behavioral Patterns*                 1961–1965†

Eiduson, Bernice T., Ph.D., *Studies of Children with Alternative Life Styles*                 1972

Ekman, Paul, Ph.D., *Communication through Nonverbal Behavior*                 1966–1972

Emde, Robert N., M.D., *Development of Affect during the First Year of Life*                 1967

Engel, George, M.D., *Psychological Processes and States of
Health and Disease*                                          1961
Ericksen, Charles W., Ph.D., *Coding and Attentional Fac-
tors in Visual Perception*                                   1964
Ervin, Frank R., M.D., *Cerebral Control of Sensory
Input*                                                  1963–1968
Escalona, Sibylle K., Ph.D., *Sensori-Motor Development
and Ego Functions*                                      1963–1972
Feather, Ben W., M.D., Ph.D., *Human Conditioning and
Perceptual Learning*                                    1963–1971
Feder, Harvey, Ph.D., *Hormonal Regulation of Behavior*      1970
Feldman, Samuel M., Ph.D., *Neuro-Behavioral Analysis of
Sensory Transmission*                                   1969–1971
Ferster, Charles B., Ph.D., *Complex Behavioral Repertoires
in Chimpanzees*                                         1963–1967
Fineman, Abraham, M.D., *Emotional Disorders of Child-
hood*                                                  1955–1958†
Fisher, Seymour, Ph.D., *Relationship of Body Emotion to
Body Reactivity*                                        1957–1961†
Flynn, John P., Ph.D., *Neural Basis of Aggression*          1965
Freedman, Daniel X., M.D., *Explorations in Psycho-
pharmacology*                                           1957–1966†
French, John R. P., Jr., Ph.D., *Interaction of Self-Identity
with the Social Environment*                                 1964
Friedel, Robert O., M.D., *CNS Phospholipid Metabolism
and Neuronal Function*                                       1970
Friedhoff, Arnold J., M.D., *Chemical Factors in Abnormal
Behavior*                                                    1961
Friedman, Stanford B., M.D., *Scheduled Behavior and
Host Resistance in Mice*                                     1962
Fuster, Joaquin M., M.D., *Cerebral Mechanism of Per-
ceptual Attention*                                          1960†
Galin, David, M.D., *Sensory and Cardiovascular Mechan-
isms in Attention*                                           1968
Gardner, Beatrice T., D. Phil., *Two-Way Communication
in Primates*                                                 1967
Gardner, Riley, Ph.D., *Origins and Implications of Cogni-
tive Organization*                                           1964
Gardner, Russell, Jr., M.D., *Investigations of Movement
during Sleep*                                                1970
Garmezy, Norman, Ph.D., *Vulnerable Children: Precursors
to Psychopathology*                                          1961

Geertz, Clifford J., Ph.D., *Comparative Studies in the Theory of Culture*                                    1964–1970

Gibson, James J., Ph.D., *Development and Test of a Theory of Perception*                                    1964–1972

Gill, Merton M., M.D., *Patient-Therapist Interaction in Psychoanalysis*                                         1963

Gillin, John P., Ph.D., *Disintegration of Sociocultural Systems*                                           1963–1972

Glick, Stanley D., Ph.D., M.D., *Drug Mechanisms in Addiction and Brain Damage*                                        1972

Goldberger, Leo, Ph.D., *Disordered Reality Contact*          1963–1968

Goldiamond, Israel, Ph.D., *Ongoing Perception and Communication*                                             1963–1967

Goldschmidt, Walter R., Ph.D., *Cultural Values and Individual Motivation*                                            1970

Goldstein, Menek, Ph.D., *Amine Metabolism and Its Relation to Mental Disease*                                      1961

Gonzalez, Richard D., Ph.D., *Comparative Psychology of Learning*                                              1963–1968

Goode, William J., Ph.D., *Control Processes in Power, Prestige, Money, Friendship Systems*                               1969

Goodenough, Donald R., Ph.D., *Studies of Dream Recall*   1963–1971

Goodwin, Donald W., M.D., *Etiological Studies of Alcoholism*                                                  1970

Gottschalk, Louis A., M.D., *Measurement Programs and Methods in Psychiatry*                                    1961–1967

Graham, Frances K., Ph.D., *Orienting and Protective Arousal Systems*                                            1964

Green, Richard, M.D., *Gender Identity: Psychologic and Biogenic Influences*                                        1969

Greenberg, Nahman, M.D., *Psychosomatic Differentiation in Infancy*                                          1961–1971†

Grosser, Bernard I., M.D., *Steroid Receptors in Brain*         1962

Haggard, Ernest A., Ph.D., *Social Isolation*                       1963

Hall, William C., Ph.D., *Structure and Function of Sensory Neocortex*                                           1971

Hargreaves, William A., Ph.D., *Behavioral Milieu in In-Patient Treatment*                                         1967

Hartman, Boyd K., M.D., *Organization of the Catecholamine Enzymes in the Brain*                                   1972

Hartmann, Ernest L., M.D., *Sleep-Dream Patterns: A Longitudinal Study*                                        1964–1969

Harvey, John A., Ph.D., *Effect of Central Nervous System
Lesions on Drug Action*                                      1964
Harvey, O. J., Ph.D., *Factors in Attitude Change*       1966–1971
Hauser, Stuart T., M.D., *Identity and Cognition: Individual and Family Studies*                                1972
Heimer, Lennart, M.D., *Light- and E-M Studies of Interneuronal Connections*                               1968–1972
Heller, Alfred, M.D., Ph.D., *Effect of CNS Lesions and
Stimulation on Brain Amines*                                 1964
Heninger, George R., M.D., *Central Neurophysiology of
the Functional Psychoses*                                    1971
Herd, James A., M.D., *Behavioral Factors in Cardiovascular Pathophysiology*                                1969
Hermann, Howard T., M.D., *Compensatory Transformations in Brain Cortex*                                  1968
Hertzig, Margaret E., M.D., *Biologic and Environmental
Influences on Behavior*                                  1968–1971
Hofer, Myron A., M.D., *Developmental Effects of Early
Maternal Separation*                                         1968
Holt, Robert R., Ph.D., *Studies in Assessing and Enhancing Ego Development*                              1962
Hooker, Evelyn, Ph.D., *Studies of Male Homosexuals*   1962–1970
Horowitz, Mardi J., M.D., *Unbidden Images: Loss of Control of Thought*                                   1964–1972
Hunt, Joseph McV., Ph.D., *Experimental Roots of Intelligence and Motivation*                             1962
Ingle, David J., Ph.D., *Neural Basis of Visual Behavior in
Lower Vertebrates*                                           1970
Jackson, Joan K., Ph.D., *Family Adaptations to Alcoholism*   1964
Jackson, Stanley W., M.D., *History of Theories and Methods of Psychoanalysis*                              1966–1971
Jaffe, Jerome H., M.D., *Pharmacological and Psychological
Factors in Drug Abuse*                                   1965–1970
Jarvik, Murray E., Ph.D., *Effects of Drugs on Memory*   1971–1972
Jones, Delmos J., Ph.D., *Impact of Urban Institutions on
Ghetto Organizations*                                        1972
Jones, Reese T., M.D., *Neuropsychology of Altered States
of Consciousness*                                            1967
Jordan, Henry A., M.D., *Experimental Analysis of Regulation of Food Intake and Hunger in Man*            1971
Kamiya, Joe, Ph.D., *Psychophysiology of Consciousness*      1968

Kandel, Eric R., M.D., *Integrative and Plastic Functions of a Simple Ganglion*                        1967

Katcher, Aaron H., M.D., *Behavioral Correlates of Cardiac Conditions*                        1963–1968

Keeler, Martin H., M.D., *Psychophysiology of Retinal Phenomena and of Psychotomimetic Drugs*                        1962–1969

Kellam, Sheppard G., M.D., *Studies of Psychopathology in Social Fields in the Community*                        1970

Kelleher, Roger T., Ph.D., *Effects of Drugs on Behavior Controlled by Aversive Stimuli*                        1964

King, Lucy J., M.D., *Effects of Drugs and Electrical Stimulation on Substrate Concentration*                        1963

Klein, Donald F., M.D., *Psychiatric Reaction Patterns to Psychotropic Drugs*                        1961–1964†

Klein, George S., Ph.D., *Cognitive Processes*                        1963–1971

Klopfer, Peter H., Ph.D., *Role of Maternal-Filial Relations in Shaping Behavior*                        1965

Knapp, Peter H., M.D., *Psychoanalytic Predictive Study of Depressive Emotion*                        1954–1959†

Knutson, Andie L., Ph.D., *The Role of Values in Health-Relevant Behavior*                        1964–1969

Koella, Werner P., Ph.D., *Role of Biogenic Amines in Organization of Sleep*                        1961–1968

Kohlberg, Lawrence, Ph.D., *Intervention and Critical Periods in Moral Development*                        1969

Komisaruk, Barry T., Ph.D., *Neuroendocrine Processes in Species-Specific Behavior*                        1969

Kornetsky, Conan, Ph.D., *Psychopharmacological Studies of Attention*                        1969

Kovach, Joseph K., Ph.D., *Heredity and Environment in Early Behavior Development*                        1970

Krall, Albert R., Ph.D., *Neurochemistry of Depression and Ion Metabolism*                        1961–1969†

Kron, Reuben E., M.D., *Experimental Investigation of Infant Sucking Behavior*                        1961–1971†

Krus, Donald M., Ph.D., *Behavioral Effects of Lysergic Acid Diethylamide and Other Drugs*                        1962–1965

Kupfer, David J., M.D., *EEG Sleep Studies in Relation to Affective Illness*                        1971

Kupferman, Irving, Ph.D., *Analysis of Learning in Aplysia Californica*                        1969

Lang, Peter J., Ph.D., *Investigation of Fear and Learned Autonomic Control*                                              1967–1972

Langner, Thomas S., Ph.D., *Psychiatric Impairment in Urban Children and Adults*                                              1972

Lehrman, Daniel S., Ph.D., *Psychobiological Studies of Behavior*                                                           1963–1972

Leiderman, P. Herbert, M.D., *Effect of Environmental Stimuli on Mental Processes*                                         1958–1963†

Lennard, Henry L., Ph.D., *Analysis of Disturbed and Therapeutic Interaction Processes*                                    1962–1972

Lenneberg, Eric H., Ph.D., *The Psychobiology of Language and Motor Coordination*                                          1959–1967†

Lesse, Henry, M.D., *Correlation of Electrical Brain Activity with Thought Processes*                                      1954–1959†

Lester, Boyd K., M.D., *Psychobiological Periodicity in Sleep and Wakefulness*                                             1961–1963†

LeVine, Robert A., Ph.D., *Cross-Cultural Study of Personality Development*                                                    1962

Levine, Seymour, Ph.D., *Hormones and Behavior*                 1963

Levinson, Daniel J., Ph.D., *Research on Personality, Role, and Social Structure*                                          1955–1971†

Levy, Edwin Z., M.D., *Residential Psychiatric Treatment for Children*                                                     1963–1967

Levy, Jerrold E., Ph.D., *Social and Cultural Meaning of Navajo Psychopathology*                                           1966–1971

Lidz, Theodore, M.D., *Schizophrenia and Family Studies*         1961

Lilly, John, M.D., *Neurophysiological, Behavioral, and Mental Concomitants of the Activities of the Brain*               1962–1967

Lipton, Morris A., M.D., Ph.D., *Biological Approaches in Psychopathology*                                                 1962–1967

Loevinger, Jane, Ph.D., *Theory and Measurement of Ego Development*                                                           1968

Loh, Horace H., Ph.D., *Neurochemical Basis of Drug Dependence*                                                               1973

London, Perry, Ph.D., *Influence of Instructions on Learning and Performance*                                             1966–1971

Luborsky, Lester B., Ph.D., *Optimal Conditions in Psychotherapy; Symptom Onset Conditions*                                  1968

Lubow, Robert E., Ph.D., *Development of Visual Pattern Perception*                                                        1963–1968

Luparello, Thomas J., M.D., *An Experimental Approach to Psychosomatic Disorders*                                          1963–1970

Lustman, Seymour L., M.D., *Normal and Pathologic Personality Development*    1961–1966

Mackworth, Norman H., Ph.D., *Perceptual Attack*    1971

Maickel, Roger, Ph.D., *Mechanism of Action of Psychoactive Drugs*    1969

Marx, Melvin H., Ph.D., *Motivation of Instrumental Behavior*    1964

Marx, Otto M., M.D., *Late-Nineteenth-Century Medical Psychology*    1968–1972

McConnell, James V., Ph.D., *Learning and Regeneration*    1963–1968

McGlothlin, William H., Ph.D., *Effects of Marijuana and Methadone on Driving Skills*    1972

McKinney, William T., Jr., M.D., *Experimental Animal Model of Depression*    1970

Melges, Frederick T., M.D., *Time Sense, Self-Concept, and Acute Mental Illness*    1967–1972

Meltzer, Herbert Y., M.D., *Biological Studies in Acutely Psychotic Patients*    1970

Mendelson, Jack H., M.D., *Metabolic and Behavioral Aspects of Alcohol Addiction*    1961–1966†

Metcalf, David R., M.D., *Behavioral and EEG Development in Infancy*    1968

Meyer, Patricia M., Ph.D., *Neocortical and Subcortical Interactions*    1967

Meyerowitz, Sanford, M.D., *Study of Psychogenic Aspects of Disease*    1961–1966†

Mintz, Norbett L., Ph.D., *Sociocultural and Familial Dynamics in Psychopathology*    1966–1972

Mirsky, Allan, Ph.D., *Studies in the Neuropsychology of Attention*    1961

Moltz, Howard, Ph.D., *Experiential and Endocrine Determinants of Maternal Behavior*    1964–1969

Mooney, William, M.D., *Experimentally Induced Ego Impairment*    1960–1965†

Musacchio, Jose M., M.D., *Regulation of Catecholamine Synthesis*    1970

Nauta, Walle J. H., M.D., Ph.D., *Experimental-Morphological Analysis of CNS Organization*    1964

Neisser, Ulric, Ph.D., *Cognitive Mechanisms*    1966–1971

Noble, Ernest P., Ph.D., M.D., *Biogenic Amines and Behavior*    1966–1969

Norton, Stata, Ph.D., *Behavior and Electrical Activity of the Brain*                                          1970

Notman, Ralph R., M.D., *Institutional Structure of the Public Mental Hospital*                               1957–1962†

Offer, Daniel, M.D., *The Modal Adolescent*                   1961–1964†

Olney, John W., M.D., *CNS Ultrastructure: Disease, Drugs, and Development*                                    1968

Overall, John E., Ph.D., *Investigation of Quantitative Approaches to Diagnosis*                              1962–1963

Patterson, Gerald R., Ph.D., *Investigation and Manipulation of Family Interaction*                            1968

Persky, Harold, Ph.D., *Endocrines, Depression, Violence, and Addiction*                                      1962

Pillard, Richard C., M.D., *Drug Effects on Induced Anxiety*                                                1967–1972

Pine, Fred J., Ph.D., *Cognitive and Motor Functions in Ego Development*                                      1962–1967

Pitts, Ferris N., Jr., M.D., *Clinical Psychiatry and Its Biochemical Correlates*                           1962–1968

Pollack, Max, Ph.D., *Neuropsychological Characterization of Schizophrenics*                                1964–1966

Prange, Arthur J., M.D., *Pharmacologic Approach to the Biology of Depression*                                1961†

Pribram, Karl H., M.D., *Neuropsychological Processes and Mechanisms*                                         1962

Quarton, Gardner C., M.D., *Effect of Thyroid and Adrenocortical Hormones on Behavior*                     1957–1963†

Raher, Jack, M.D., *Intercorrelations between Affect and Adrenal Activity*                                  1962–1967

Rechtschaffen, Allan, Ph.D., *Psychology and Physiology of Sleep*                                             1962

Reichsman, Franz, M.D., *Relationships of Behavior and Psychologic Adaptation*                              1956–1964†

Reite, Martin L., M.D., *Psychobiological Development in Monkeys*                                             1971

Reivich, Ronald S., M.D., *Multi-System Analysis of Psychotropic Drug Action*                               1967–1972

Robins, Eli, M.D., *Metabolic (Biochemical) Investigations of Psychiatric Disease*                          1961–1963

Robins, Lee N., Ph.D., *Epidemiology of Achievement and Psychiatric Status*                                   1970

Rock, Irvin, Ph.D., *Adaptation to Experimentally Altered Stimulation*    1967

Roffwarg, Howard P., M.D., *Physiology and Psychophysiology of Sleep and Dreaming*    1962

Rosenberg, Seymour, Ph.D., *Studies in Verbal Communication*    1968

Rosenblum, Leonard A., Ph.D., *Maternal Behavior and Infant Attachment*    1964–1972

Rosner, Burton S., Ph.D., *Psychophysiology of Sensory Function in Men*    1964–1969

Rossi, Alice E., Ph.D., *Family and Career Role Expectations*    1964–1969

Rothenberg, Albert, M.D., *Studies in the Creative Process*    1964

Rowland, Vernon, M.D., *Electrophysiologic Response in Perception and Learning*    1955†

Rubin, Robert T., M.D., *Psychoneuroendocrine Studies of Sleep in Man*    1972

Ruff, George E., M.D., *Stress Produced by Experimental Isolation*    1959–1964†

Sachar, Edward J., M.D., *Psychoendocrine Studies of Depressive Illness*    1964

Sander, Louis W., M.D., *The Adaptive Process in Infant Environment Interaction*    1963

Sanford, R. Nevitt, Ph.D., *Social Innovation: Inquiring and Action on Aggression*    1969

Sapira, Joseph D., M.D., *Alterations of Epinephrine Secretory Rates in Man*    1970–1971

Satterfield, James H., M.D., *Neurophysiological Correlates of Behavior*    1961–1966†

Schanberg, Saul M., M.D., Ph.D., *Neurotropic Drug Effects on Biogenic Amine Metabolism*    1968

Schiavi, Raul C., M.D., *CNS Control of Gonadal Function and Sexual Behavior*    1965–1966

Schuster, Charles R., Ph.D., *Psychopharmacology of Drug Abuse*    1971

Scott, John W., Jr., Ph.D., *Olfactory Input to the Hypothalamus*    1971

Segal, Sydney J., Ph.D., *Imagery and Perception: Parameters of Reality Testing*    1971–1972

Seiden, Lewis S., Ph.D., *Brain Amines and Conditioned Behavior*    1967

Serafetinides, Eustace A., M.D., Ph.D., *Bioelectrical Neuro-psychiatry of Consciousness*                  1967–1972

Shapiro, David, Ph.D., *Instrumental Properties of ANS Functions*                  1963

Shaw, Evelyn, Ph.D., *Environmental Modifiers of Behavioral Development*                  1963

Shellenberger, M. Kent, Ph.D., *Brain Function—Drug Mechanisms: Chemistry, Physiology*                  1972

Simmons, Roberta G., Ph.D., *Self-Image Development in Children*                  1970

Skinner, B. F., Ph.D., *Behavioral Analysis of Cultural Practices*                  1964

Snapper, Arthur G., Ph.D., *Behavioral and Cardiac Effects of Aversive Control*                  1972

Snyder, Solomon H., M.D., *Metabolism of Biogenic Amines*                  1966

Spear, Norman E., Ph.D., *Memory and Retrieval Failure in the Rat*                  1970

Spence, Donald P., Ph.D., *Verbal and Autonomic Studies of Clinical Judgments*                  1961

Spohn, Herbert E., Ph.D., *Behavioral Mechanisms of Drug Action in Schizophrenia*                  1971

Stechler, Gerald, Ph.D., *Experimental Analysis of Operant Discrimination*                  1962–1972

Stewart, Mark A., M.D., *Enzyme Synthesis in the Developing Nervous System*                  1961–1971†

Stilson, Donald W., Ph.D., *Neurophysiological Models of Elementary Behaviors*                  1969

Stein, Donald G., Ph.D., *Recovery of Function in the CNS*                  1972

Stein, Marvin, M.D., *Clinical and Experimental Studies of Bronchial Asthma*                  1956–1963†

Stein, Morris I., Ph.D., *Studies in Creativity and Assessment*                  1962

Stock, Dorothy, Ph.D., *Studies in the Therapeutic Interaction*                  1961–1964

Stone, Eric A., Ph.D., *Behavioral and Neurochemical Effects of Severe Stress*                  1971

Stoyva, Johann M., Ph.D., *Bioelectric Information Feedback in Therapy*                  1969

Straumanis, John J., Jr., M.D., *Evoked Cerebral Responses in Psychiatric Disorders*                  1966–1971

Stross, Lawrence, M.D., *Ego States and Varieties of Consciousness*                                                         1962–1967

Studt, Elliot T., D.S.W., *Re-Socialization of Offenders
through Parole*                                                     1964–1969

Tanguay, Peter E., M.D., *CNS Maturity in Infantile
Autism: Study of Sleep EEG*                                        1970

Taylor, Anna N., Ph.D., *Central Mechanisms in Endo-
crine Responses to Stress*                                         1972

Thiessen, Delbert D., Ph.D., *Single-Gene Substitution and
Behavior in Mice*                                                  1968–1972

Thompson, Richard F., Ph.D., *Learning and the Central
Nervous System*                                                    1962

Thurman, Ronald G., Ph.D., *Mixed-Function Oxidation
and Intermediary Metabolism*                                       1972

Titchener, James L., M.D., *Emotional Phenomena in Can-
cer Patients*                                                       1955–1960†

Tobach, Ethel, Ph.D., *Vertebrate Emotional Behavior—
Phylogeny and Ontogeny*                                            1964

Tomkins, Silvan S., Ph.D., *Studies in Affect and Cognition*       1964

Uhlenhuth, Eberhard H., M.D., *States of Subjective Dis-
tress and their Motivation*                                        1962–1968

Uttal, William R., Ph.D., *Neurophysiological Basis of
Sensation and Perception*                                          1971

Vaillant, George E., M.D., *Follow-Up of Normal Adults,
Schizophrenics, and Addicts*                                       1968–1971

Valenstein, Elliot S., Ph.D., *Physiology of Motivation and
Learning*                                                          1963–1971

Vandenberg, Steven G., Ph.D., *Five-Year Study of Neo-
nate Twins*                                                        1962–1967

Vernadakis, Antonia O., Ph.D., *Physiology and Pharmacology of the Developing CNS*                                         1969

Walker, Edward L., Ph.D., *Problems in the Memory-
Storage Process and the Determinants of Choice*                    1964

Walzer, Stanley, M.D., *Variation in Behavior with Sex-
Chromosome Aberrations*                                            1968

Warren, Roland L., Ph.D., *Community Structure and
Planned Social Change*                                             1964

Waxler, Nancy E., Ph.D., *Families and Schizophrenia:
Studies of Deviance*                                               1968

Weiner, Herbert, M.D., *Studies of Evoked Potentials in
Animals and Men*                                                   1962–1965

# Appendix B: Members of the Mental Health Career Investigator Selection Committee, Mental Health Research Career Award Committee, and/or Research Scientist Development Review Committee

|  | Tenure |
|---|---|
| Dr. Alan Gregg (Chairman, 1953–1956) | 1953–1956 |
| Dr. Horace Magoun | 1953–1954 |
| Dr. John D. Benjamin | 1953–1956 |
| Dr. Henry W. Brosin | 1953–1956 |
| Dr. David Shakow | 1953–1957 |
| Dr. Robert B. Livingston | 1954–1957 |
| Dr. S. Howard Armstrong, Jr. | 1955–1959 |
| Dr. Lawrence C. Kolb (Chairman, 1959–1960) | 1955–1960 |
| Dr. John Romano (Chairman, 1956–1959; 1960–1961) | 1956–1961 |
| Dr. Max M. Levin | 1957–1961 |
| Dr. Paul D. MacLean | 1957–1961 |
| Dr. Jerome D. Frank | 1959–1961; 1968–1969 |
| Dr. Morton F. Reiser (Chairman, 1961–1963) | 1959–1963 |
| Dr. Kenneth E. Clark | 1960–1964 |
| Dr. John A. Clausen | 1960–1964 |
| Dr. Herbert S. Gaskill | 1960–1964 |
| Dr. John W. Mason | 1960–1963 |
| Dr. Louis C. Lasagna | 1961–1965 |
| Dr. David A. Hamburg (Chairman, 1963–1965) | 1961–1965 |
| Dr. Frederic G. Worden | 1961–1966; 1971–1975 |
| Dr. I. Charles Kaufman | 1962–1964 |
| Dr. Benjamin D. Paul | 1962–1963 |
| Dr. Daniel Miller | 1962–1966 |
| Dr. L. Joseph Stone | 1962–1966 |

| | |
|---|---|
| Dr. Marvin Stein (Chairman, 1965–1967) | 1963–1967 |
| Dr. John I. Lacey | 1964–1965 |
| Dr. Harold L. Wilensky | 1964–1967 |
| Dr. Ernest A. Haggard (Chairman, 1967–1968) | 1964–1968 |
| Dr. Kenneth MacCorquodale | 1964–1968 |
| Dr. Alfred H. Stanton | 1964–1968 |
| Dr. Austin H. Riesen | 1964–1969 |
| Dr. Walle J. H. Nauta | 1966–1968 |
| Dr. Guy E. Swanson | 1966–1968 |
| Dr. H. Enger Rosvold | 1966–1969 |
| Dr. Robert S. Wallerstein (Chairman, 1968–1970) | 1966–1970 |
| Dr. Albert J. Stunkard | 1966–1970 |
| Dr. Alberta E. Siegel | 1966–1970 |
| Dr. Samuel Eiduson | 1966–1970 |
| Dr. Herbert Weiner | 1967–1971 |
| Dr. Howard E. Freeman | 1967–1971 |
| Dr. Nicholas J. Giarman | 1968 |
| Dr. Kenneth B. Little | 1968–1969 |
| Dr. Edward L. Walker (Chairman, 1970–1972) | 1968–1972 |
| Dr. Jacob Cohen | 1968–1972 |
| Dr. Akira Horita | 1969–1973 |
| Dr. Daniel X. Freedman | 1969–1973 |
| Dr. Richard F. Thompson | 1969–1973 |
| Dr. Joseph C. Speisman | 1969–1973 |
| Dr. Albert J. Silverman (Chairman, 1972–1974) | 1970–1974 |
| Dr. John P. Flynn | 1970–1974 |
| Dr. Arthur Yuwiler | 1970–1974 |
| Dr. Albert McQueen | 1971–1975 |
| Dr. Lucy Rau Ferguson | 1971–1975 |
| Dr. John E. Overall | 1972–1976 |
| Dr. Edith Neimark | 1972–1976 |
| Dr. Lyman C. Wynne | 1972–1976 |

# Appendix C: The Selection Process

How is a Research Development Program awardee selected? The Review Committee's decision process is exceptionally impressive to those who have observed it directly or who have participated in it; it seems mysterious to those who have not been closely associated with it. There is therefore some virtue in a brief description of the character and sequence of actions that lead to a decision concerning the scientific merits of the proposal. (It should be emphasized that the Committee's actions are advisory only; they recommend to Institute staff that an application warrants approval but do not direct the staff to make an award.)

The Committee normally consists of 13 scientists who are not on the NIMH staff. Its meetings are attended by one to six NIMH staff members, depending on the subject of the proposal. Scientists on the Committee are selected by the Assistant Secretary for Health (on the recommendation of the Director of NIMH) to represent as nearly as possible the range of scientific issues likely to require Committee review. Members serve for four years and a new chairman is chosen every one or two years. Psychiatry tends to be the most heavily represented discipline on the Committee, with three or four members at any one time. Other areas commonly represented include biochemistry or neurochemistry, psychopharmacology, neurophysiology and neuroanatomy, clinical psychology, experimental psychology, developmental psychology, sociology, anthropology, and statistics. Normally, three members retire each year and are replaced in such a manner that the work load of Committee members is as nearly balanced as possible.

The review process begins when a complete application is received in NIMH and assigned to the Research Scientist Development Section. A complete application contains, as a minimum: a complete plan for five years of research and training (if training is appropriate); a curriculum vitae; a list of the candidate's publications and a sample of reprints; a statement of the institution's program of relevant research; and a statement of the role the individual candidate is expected to play in the institution's program. This material can represent as few as 40 to 50 pages or as many as 1,000 or more.

The Executive Secretary of the Research Scientist Development Award Section then chooses one member of the Committee to be the primary reader and representative for each candidate on the basis of the nature of the proposal and the scientific background of the Committee member. One secondary reader (although occasionally as many as three) is also assigned to each proposal at the same time. The primary and secondary readers are then sent the entire proposal and copies of all reprints and letters of reference. The other members of the Committee receive copies of the proposal and letters of reference.

Before a meeting, a Committee member might receive two or three complete sets of materials for which he will be the primary reader, three to five complete sets of materials for which he will be secondary reader, and perhaps 20 to 30 other proposals not accompanied by supplementary material.

A primary or secondary reader is expected to master the content of the proposal as well as all other supplementary material. With many proposals, the material received is sufficient. In many cases, however, it is not. A genuine understanding of the proposal may require reading other publications by the candidate or the publications of other individuals or groups on which the candidate has based his proposal. These duties may take from three to six days of work before each of the four meetings per year. (Committee members are not compensated financially for this phase of the review process—their time is donated.)

It is sometimes necessary to obtain expert opinion outside the Committee itself. This is sometimes done by the NIMH staff when the need can be anticipated, but it is often done by the primary reader who knows the one or two men in the world who can provide the requisite information and judgment. When necessary, such an outside expert is invited to serve as an ad hoc member of the Committee through all or part of the process of consideration and decision.

A proposal considered in depth by one to three Committee members is listed on the agenda of the next meeting for preliminary consideration. When it is considered, the primary reader explains the proposal's content to all other Committee members. (Committee members from the same institution as the candidate are never present during any aspect of the proposal's consideration; in order to ensure that scientific merit is the only criterion of judgment, committee members who might have any conflict of interest are not present during deliberations.) It is this phase of the review process that makes service on the Committee interesting and exciting. Members pay with their own time and work for the privilege of hearing others present the intricacies and prospects for the advancing knowledge in areas somewhat removed from their own. Such expositions are uniformly competent and frequently brilliant.

When the primary reader has made his presentation, secondary readers contribute their individual comments and degrees of agreement or disagreement. This is followed by a general discussion by the whole Committee. In the process of this discussion, consensus is usually reached. Four possible recommendations are most common at this stage: rejection, withdrawal, approval without site visit, and deferred action pending a site visit. A proposal may be rejected for any number of reasons ranging from a negative evaluation of the proposal to a decision that this particular form of support is not likely to affect appreciably the course and progress of the research. Occasionally, a candidate will be asked if he wishes to withdraw the proposal, either because it was not adequately formulated or because it was inappropriate for this particular program. A third possible outcome at this stage is to recommend for approval without site visit. This exceedingly rare decision occurs only when the merits of the proposal and the candidate are unquestionable and when no positive purpose can be envisioned for the site visit. The most frequent decision is to defer further action until after a site visit.

If a site visit is projected, the Committee members usually outline rather precisely what information concerning the candidate, the proposal, or the setting the site visitors are to obtain. The members then suggest to the Executive Secretary which individuals might have the competence, knowledge, and skill to acquire the necessary information and make the requisite judgments. A site visit team is composed of three to five persons, including one or two Committee members. Usually, one member of the Committee is given major responsibility for arranging the visit and reporting its results. The site visit committee may then by supplemented by one to three outside scientists, depending on the complexity of the proposal and the range of expertise required to deal with it. The Executive Secretary of the Committee is almost always a member of the site-visit team unless his work load on the Committee is too heavy.

Usually the site visit is carried out before the next meeting of the Research Scientist Development Review Committee, and the proposal is listed for final action at that meeting. At that time, the reviewing process is almost identical to the preliminary review except that studying a proposal for a second time requires less effort on the part of Committee members, and the site visit report is available as well. In addition, the Committee members who made the site visit are available to report on its progress, outcome, and findings and to answer Committee members' questions. Normally, at the end of this second complete review of the proposal, the Committee members vote to recommend either approval or disapproval. If the vote is for disapproval, one Committee member is assigned to write a complete report on the proposal, its discussion, and the reasons for disapproval. If the majority votes to recommend approval, the process is identical, except that the report states the reasons for approval, and each member of the Committee is asked to assign a priority number to the proposal on a scale of one to five. The average of this priority assignment can then be used as a guide by the NIMH staff in making awards when there are insufficient funds to support all approved applications. Finally, if there is a split vote, two summaries are prepared by two different members of the Committee, one summarizing the majority opinion and the other the minority opinion.

# Appendix D: Program Administrators

Appendix D lists NIMH officials associated with the Research Development Program. Dates refer to period of association as of early 1973.

*Institute Directors*

| | |
|---|---|
| Robert B. Felix, M.D. | 1952–1964 |
| Stanley F. Yolles, M.D. | 1964–1970 |
| Bertram S. Brown, M.D. | 1970 to present |

*Division and/or Branch Directors*

Chief, Research Grants and Fellowships Branch
| | |
|---|---|
| John C. Eberhart, Ph.D. | 1952–1954 |
| Philip Sapir | 1954–1964 |

Chief, Training and Manpower Resources Branch
| | |
|---|---|
| Eli A. Rubinstein, Ph.D. | 1964–1966 |

Director, Division of Manpower and Training Programs
| | |
|---|---|
| Eli A. Rubinstein, Ph.D. | 1966–1967 |
| Raymond J. Balester, Ph.D. | 1967–1968 |

Chief, Behavioral Sciences Training Branch
| | |
|---|---|
| Joseph C. Speisman, Ph.D. | 1966–1968 |

|  |  |
|---|---|
| George Ham, M.D. | 1968–1969 |
| Thomas F. Plaut, Ph.D. | 1969–1971 |
| Bernard Bandler, M.D. | 1971–1972 |

*Chief, Behavioral Sciences Training Branch*

|  |  |
|---|---|
| Bert E. Boothe, Ph.D. | 1968–1971 |
| F. Neil Waldrop, M.D. | 1972–1973 |

*Chief, Behavioral Sciences Training Branch*

|  |  |
|---|---|
| Fred Elmadjian, Ph.D. | 1971–1973 |

*Director, Division of Extramural Research Programs*

|  |  |
|---|---|
| Louis A. Wienckowski, Ph.D. | 1973 to present |

*Section Directors*
   *Chief, Research Fellowships Section*

|  |  |
|---|---|
| Bert E. Boothe, Ph.D. | 1961–1968 |

   *Chief, Research Scientist Development Section*

|  |  |
|---|---|
| Mary R. Haworth, Ph.D. | 1968 to present |

*Executive Secretaries*
   *Fellowship and Career Investigator Program*

|  |  |
|---|---|
| Philip Sapir | 1954–1957 |
| Bert E. Boothe, Ph.D. | 1957–1963 |

   *Research Career Program*

|  |  |
|---|---|
| Betty H. Pickett, Ph.D. | 1963–1966 |

   *Research Development Program*

|  |  |
|---|---|
| Mary R. Haworth, Ph.D. | 1967 to present |

*Grants Assistants and Secretaries*
   *Grants Assistant*

|  |  |
|---|---|
| Marjorie Cross | 1957 to present |

   *Secretaries*

|  |  |
|---|---|
| Justice Davidson | 1963–1967 |
| Jeannette Raley | 1963 to present |

   *Technical Assistant*

|  |  |
|---|---|
| Jeannette Raley | 1970 to present |

# References

Albee, G. W. The uncertain future of clinical psychology. *American Psychologist*, 1970, **25**, 1071–1080.

Asher, R. Talking sense. *Lancet*, 1959, **2**, 417.

Group for the Advancement of Psychiatry. *The Recruitment and Training of the Research Psychiatrist*, 1967, Report No. 65.

Ham, C. Reintegration of psychoanalysis into teaching. *American Journal of Psychiatry*, 1961, **117**, 877.

Hamburg, D. A. (Ed.) *Psychiatry as a Behavioral Science*. Englewood Cliffs, N.J.: Prentice-Hall, 1970.

Freedman, D. X. "Can we put research to use?" Keynote address presented March 1972 at the 17th Annual Conference, VA Cooperative Studies in Mental Health and Behavioral Sciences, Jointly Sponsored by the VA and the Eastern Missouri Psychiatric Society.

Offer, D., Freedman, D. X., and Offer, J. The psychiatrist as researcher. In D. Offer and D. X. Freedman (Eds.) *Modern Psychiatry and Clinical Research: Essays in Honor of Roy R. Grinker, Sr.* New York: Basic Books, 1972.

Romano, J. Basic orientation and education of the medical student. *Journal of the American Medical Association*, 1950, **143**, 409.

Romano, J. Teaching of psychiatry to medical students. *Lancet*, 1961, **2**, 93.

Rothman, T. In P. H. Hock and J. Zubin (Eds.) *The Future of Psychiatry*. New York: Grune & Stratton, 1962.

Shakow, D. "The education of the mental health researcher: Encouraging potential development in man." Third Verstermark Memorial Lecture, Presented October 6, 1971, at the National Center for Mental Health Services, Training, and Research.

Shepherd, M. A critical appraisal of contemporary psychiatry. *Comprehensive Psychiatry*, 1971, **12**, 302–320.

# Index